W9-AYZ-820

REGULATING HOSPITAL COSTS:
The Development of Public Policy

REGULATING HOSPITAL COSTS:
The Development of Public Policy

David S. Abernethy

and

David A. Pearson

AUPHA PRESS
Ann Arbor, Michigan • Washington, D.C.
1979

Copyright © 1979 by The Regents of The University of Michigan.
Printed in the United States of America. All rights reserved. This
book or parts thereof may not be reproduced in any form without
written permission of the publisher.

Library of Congress Cataloging in Publication Data

Abernethy, David S
  Regulating hospital costs.

  Bibliography: p.
  Includes indexes.
  1. Hospitals — Cost control — Law and legislation — United
States. 2. Hospitals — United States — Cost control. 3. Hospitals
United States — Cost of operation. I. Pearson, David, 1935–
joint author. II. Title.
KF3825.5.A93   344'.73'0321   79-9227
ISBN 0-914904-36-1
ISBN 0-914904-37-X pbk.

AUPHA PRESS
One DuPont Circle
Washington, D.C.
and
The School of Public Health
The University of Michigan
Ann Arbor, Michigan
1979

To Rodney and Elizabeth Abernethy
and for
Karin and Mark Pearson

About the Authors

David S. Abernethy

David S. Abernethy, M.P.H. is Minority Staff Associate, Subcommittee on Health and the Environment, Committee on Interstate and Foreign Commerce, United States House of Representatives. He has been involved in the design of legislation concerning hospital cost containment, health planning, health maintenance organizations, regulation of pharmaceuticals, and drug abuse treatment and control. Mr. Abernethy is the former Administrator, Haight-Ashbury Medical Clinic, San Francisco. He received his M.P.H. in Health Services Administration from Yale University.

David A. Pearson

David A. Pearson, Ph.D. is Associate Dean for Public Health and Associate Professor in the Department of Epidemiology and Public Health, Yale University School of Medicine and in the University's Institution for Social and Policy Studies. Previously he was Director, Office of Regional Activities, Yale University School of Medicine. From 1961 to 1968, he held various positions in the U.S. Public Health Service including Director, Health Economics Program, National Center for Health Services Research. He coauthored *Dynamics of Health and Disease,* and is completing work on a manuscript dealing with the regional organization of health services. He has contributed numerous articles in such areas as health economics, the epidemiology of health services, and policy issues associated with the organization and delivery of health services.

Contents

III THE CONGRESSIONAL RESPONSE

IV ASSESSMENT

11   Conclusion

Tables

Foreword

The attempt of the 95th Congress to pass some sort of hospital cost containment legislation ended with more of a whimper than a bang, lost in a welter of bills at the end of the session. Hardly had the interment taken place when the *Wall Street Journal* of October 24, 1978 predicted that new federal cost containment legislation was likely to reemerge in the form of well-defined proposals in the winter of 1979 or early 1980.

This book, which reviews the 1978 activity, has definite relevance to any general consideration of future government efforts to control hospital costs. In addition, it appropriately provides a documentation of previous efforts.

Any such consideration of a recent legislative effort to contain hospital costs must be based on one assumption and at least two factors which appear as themes threading through this history, and which will probably be reappearing in future legislative proposals. The basic assumption is that the availability of federal monies have included, do include, and ever will include some degree of federal control. The two issues in question then, fall under public accountability—how much and what kind of control will be exerted and social engineering—how many controls will be imposed to achieve the goals of the legislation.

The importance of this seemingly arbitrary split between the two main thrusts of most federal legislation is that it accents the fact that social engineering costs money, however valid or relevant are its aims. It is not free. Such an identification is critical, then, in a legislative attempt to contain costs, and certainly in an attempt not to increase them. Because much of this social engineering is labeled in innocuous or publicly acceptable terms such as accessibility, equity, equal opportunity, or bilingual education, many of the economic implications of such controls are not isolated and discussed.

In other words, social engineering is signified not in a perjorative sense, but to distinguish it from the area of public accountability. Social engineering represents the tendency to use payment methods to change either the organization of or the places where the services are delivered, as well as to define the amount and number of the services provided. Indeed, some of the most recent federal legislation in health has attempted to make up for the lack of such provisions in previous legislation.

The legislation reviewed in this book contains both the aspects of public accountability and of social engineering. The main purpose of the law was to be to contain hospital costs. There was a minimal attempt to change the system or to redefine the role of system components or even cost containment for components of the system other than hospitals. There was, however, an effort to redistribute relative income among hospital workers, particularly those nonprofessional workers who would likely be members of some kind of union. The pass-through on ceilings for negotiated labor contracts may be a most desirable social goal; that is not the question. What is the question here is whether an escape clause, and its subsequent ripple effect on other employees, might have resulted in situations that are equally as undesirable as have been experienced with reimbursement based on "reasonable cost." It should be noted that the one state with some experience in such pass-throughs (New York) specifically requested a waiver for the pass-through provision.

In the past, the health industry has been most fortunate in the balance of these two types of controls imposed by the federal government in return for its largesse. Many believe, on the other hand, that not enough change was legislated along with the money, and a strong case can be made that many of the health delivery problems of today are due to earlier failures to change the system. The Hill-Burton Act exerted few controls over the hospital beneficiaries of capital contributions, other than exacting the guarantee that they continue to operate as hospitals the institutions built with federal monies. Accountability was mainly concerned with the compliance to federal standards of the building itself, standards which were certainly not onerous and, indeed, were in the best interests of patient safety. The social engineering aspect of legislation was borne mainly by the states which were, for the first time, directed to derive some kind of state hospital plan based on a very loose interpretation of the regional hospital "system."

In Medicare and, to a lesser extent, Medicaid, the controls, again, were minimal because of a blind faith in that exotic phrase, "reasonable costs," upon which payments were to be based. Although utilization review was required immediately by Medicare and eventually theoretically by Medicaid, it never really changed the system because it seemed to have little effect on influencing the way providers performed. Indeed, the length of stay increased rather dramatically in nonfederal short-term general and other special hospitals from the level of approximately 7.6 days before Medicaid to 8.4 days in 1968. It was only in 1977 that the length of stay reverted to the level of 7.6 days experienced in 1960. Many believe that one of the problems with the Medicare and Medicaid legislation was a lack of social engineering, with little attempt to make medical care institutions more accountable to, or responsive to, the needs of the populations they served.

The two factors which seem to affect the ability of the cost containment legislation discussed in this book to become law were, first, an uncomfortable feeling about the federal government's previous lack of ability to control medical care costs altogether and, in particular, hospital costs. The Office of Planning, Evaluation and Legislation report on the effectiveness of PSROs was not at all encouraging. Health Systems Agencies created by P.L. 93–641 were too new and, consequently, had no track record to indicate whether or not they could affect costs better than their predecessors in the Comprehensive Health Planning Program. Although this issue did not arise, except in some selected hearings and publicity releases, the faith that one could put in the various state governments which had undertaken cost control seemed to be more favorable.

The second factor that emerged in the overall assessments of the specific legislation and, again, this did not appear too often in the formal history of the legislation, was the feeling of discomfort with the state of the art regarding just how anyone could contain hospital costs without negatively influencing quality or accessibility. The Harris poll of April 1978 revealed that this uncertainty was certainly shared by the public which, at this time, seemed to want its cake and, further, seemed to want the bakery within reasonable travel distance from home. The public, then, has failed to deal with the trade-offs between some changes in the accessibility of certain services and their cost. It is, therefore, impossible to create much of a public constituency to support a legislative effort which implicitly deals with the cost, accountability, and quality conundrum.

One issue is clear; all parties involved, government, providers, payers, scholars, and the public, must become more knowledgeable about the issues involved in hospital cost containment if any different kind of a history is to be written on the subject. This book, therefore, represents a basic knowledge base for all parties identified above.

John D. Thompson, *Professor of Public Health (Hospital Administration) Department of Epidemiology and Public Health Yale University Medical School*

Preface

There is little question that inflation in health and medical care costs, particularly hospital costs, is a serious problem. First, there are many signs that this country is experiencing difficulty in financing its health care system. Second, the system is perceived by some to be an inefficient producer of its ultimate goal—better health. Also there is concern that the costs are outstripping the benefits. And finally, there are other competing social goals to which national resources could be committed if health care costs could be controlled.

The causes of health care inflation are many, but research findings indicate that the open-ended third party reimbursement system is a major factor. With more than 94 percent of hospital costs paid by public and private third party payers, consumers have come to accept a higher style of care than needed and providers have been allowed to follow powerful incentives towards higher quantity and higher intensity care with questions raised about the efficacy of such actions.

The Hospital Cost Containment bill of 1977 has sought to impose a set of relatively arbitrary controls on this highly complex and little understood system to reverse or curb present trends. The legislation has met with controversy for four reasons. First, health care is widely accepted as a desirable social goal. Second, the causes of inflation are open to question. Third, a great deal of bias exists against greater federal regulation. And fourth, the limited data base upon which decisions are being made contributes to the difficulty in analyzing the impact the proposed act may have on the health care system.

This book is a descriptive and qualitatively analytical discussion of the policy struggle in Congress over the Hospital Cost Containment Act. Against a background of severe and unceasing inflation in health care costs, an understanding of this struggle provides a perspective on the probability that health care inflation will ever be brought under control. We intend to provide that perspective in a variety of ways. Available statistical indicators are presented to identify the dimensions of the problems. Various theories which have been advanced to explain inflation in the health care industry are presented and discussed, followed by a discussion of previous efforts to control health care inflation. The theories of inflation are stressed because we contend that the confusion and lack of understanding of why health care costs are inflating have contributed significantly to the difficulty surrounding passage of the Hospital Cost Containment Act. Similarly we discuss the efficacy and fairness of previous control efforts and conclude that they had a sizeable impact on judgments made by Congress about the value of the proposed act.

After providing a theoretical base, we trace the progress of the legislation through Congress, describing the players, their motivations, and their impact, providing an example of how this nation decides between competing goals and conflicting viewpoints. In this respect, the Hospital Cost Containment Act is especially interesting to analyze, since the subject matter of concern is health—a commodity which our society believes should be available to all.

David S. Abernethy
David A. Pearson

Acknowledgements

This book would not have been possible without the interest and assistance provided to us by the Honorable Tim Lee Carter, M.D., Congressman from the Fifth District of Kentucky and Ranking Minority Member of the Subcommittee on Health and the Environment. To this warm and generous individual, we owe a great deal of thanks.

Many persons provided guidance, assistance or information for which we are most grateful. In particular, Frances dePeyster and Douglas Francisco of Congressman Carter's staff deserve special thanks and acknowledgement. Karen Nelson, Robert Crane, and William Corr of the Majority Staff of the Subcommittee on Health and the Environment are gratefully acknowledged for providing information and counsel.

At Yale, we wish especially to acknowledge Arthur J. Viseltear, Stephen S. Mick, and John D. Thompson for sharing their knowledge and providing us with assistance and friendship. To Vera Wardlaw and Betsy Francisco we give our gratitude for their superb skills as editors and typists.

DSA
DAP

New Haven, Connecticut
November 21, 1978

I | The Setting

1 | A Perspective On Inflation In Health Care Costs

"The medical crisis ... is purely and simply a crisis of cost. The inflationary rise in medical costs is the key concern of congressmen and consumers, a fundamental political and economic fact of life for both."[1]

Introduction

National health care expenditures more than quadrupled between 1965 and 1975 and the annual expenditure for 1977 is estimated at $162.6 billion, an increase of 12 percent over the previous year. During the same period the Gross National Product only doubled, thereby increasing the health care share of the GNP from 5.9 to 8.8 percent; per capita spending for health increased from $197.75 to an estimated $736.92.[2]

It has become almost a cliché to begin an inquiry on the health care delivery system with an accounting of such figures. Paper after paper recounts the statistics of inflation while politicians, labor and business leaders, hospital administrators, doctors, and policy analysts express their profound concern in speeches, articles, and statements. Furthermore, public opinion polls indicate that rising health care costs are among the top three domestic concerns of the American people, ranking ahead of rising energy costs.

The Carter administration attempted to answer this concern by introducing the Hospital Cost Containment Act, and struggled with the Congress for over a year to pass this legislation. Given the seemingly widespread concern over inflation in health care costs, it is sometimes difficult to comprehend why the administration has had little success in securing passage of this legislation. Clearly, the administration's difficulty could lead an observer to ask if the hospital industry was truly powerful enough to successfully block congressional approval of the bill. One might also be likely to ask if the cost containment methodology included in the bill was thought to be inequitable or unworkable.

Is Inflation a Problem?

Inflation in the costs of direct health care delivery is not necessarily bad. There is no economic rule stating that 5, or 9, or even 12 percent of GNP is the appropriate amount society should spend on health care delivery. Health care is widely accepted as a necessary social good, one to which each member of a society is entitled. One need look no farther than the passage of Medicare and Medicaid in 1965, or the $4.1 billion spent for hospital construction by the Hill-Burton program between 1947 and 1974,[3] for evidence of the importance placed on health care in this country.

Inflation in health care costs becomes a problem when: (1) it outstrips society's ability to pay, (2) the services which are delivered are not perceived to be provided in an efficient fashion, (3) the benefits accruing to society are not perceived to be worth the costs, and (4) the cost of providing the present type and amount of services is perceived to preclude the purchase or provision of other goods or services of greater benefit.

In assessing how this society answers the questions implied by these four points, a good starting point is an analysis provided by Fuchs,[4] who points out that there are two common fallacies often voiced by those involved in health care: first, resources are no longer scarce, and second, health is the most important goal. He refutes these points by explaining, in the case of the first statement:

> the fundamental fact remains that even if all ... imperfections were eliminated total output would still fall short of the amount people would like to have. Resources would still be short in the sense that choices would have to be made.

In the case of the second statement, he states that:

> Some of those in the health field recognize that we cannot satisfy all wants, but they seem to believe that health is more important than all other goals and therefore questions of scarcity and allocation are not applicable in this area. It requires only a casual study of human behavior to reveal the fallacy of this position. Every day in manifold ways people make choices that affect health and it is clear that they frequently place a higher value on satisfying other wants: e.g., smoking, overeating, careless driving, failure to take medicine, etc.

From this intuitively satisfying analysis, the question of whether inflation in health care costs is inappropriate in and of itself can be restated in terms of scarce resources and competing goals. Therefore, if society finds that inflation is outstripping its ability to pay for health and medical care services, it can be concluded that the mechanism for allocating resources to health is not working properly because too many scarce resources are going to health to the detriment of other present commitments. There is a great deal of evidence that this society is having significant difficulty in funding its health care delivery system.

Can We Afford Our Health Care System?

Perhaps the most famous statement of a business leader on the problem of paying for health care delivery is that of Victor Zink, Director, Employee Benefits and Services for General Motors, who pointed out that GM first negotiated Blue Cross and Blue Shield coverage for its workers 25 years ago, at a time when the total income of all Blue Cross and Blue Shield plans was approximately $455 million. By 1975, GM alone paid $735 million for basic health coverage for its U.S. workers. GM's annualized health care costs rose from $735 million in 1975 to $825 million in 1976 for a total of about $1,700 a year for every employee on its payroll. "Another way of looking at it is that the Blue Cross and Blue Shield Plans—if considered together—are by far [GM's] largest single supplier. Metropolitan Life is second, and United States Steel is a distant third."[5]

Additional statements by business and labor leaders further underscore the difficulty this country is having in meeting its health care bill.[6] Charles L. Glass of Eastern Airlines noted that, "except for the cost of fuel, I am unaware of any single cost element which has escalated as much as medical insurance costs." The 25 percent annual increase experienced by Eastern Airlines occurred during a time when the benefit package remained fairly stable.

Various union leaders testified to the difficulty in retaining the same level of benefits they have enjoyed in the past in the face of acute inflation in health care costs:

> Just to maintain our current level of health benefits requires labor negotiators to seek annual increases of 14% or more, the rate at which health costs are increasing. Some unions that administer their own health and welfare funds [instead of the company providing health insurance coverage] have been forced to reduce benefits until such time as they can negotiate increased health benefits [usually specific dollar amounts per hour worked] from the employer. (Joseph R. Ferrara, Area Director of Region 9 of the United Automobile Workers)

When we negotiate the package deal, 70-75% invariably winds up going into health and welfare because of inflation, and it's pretty tough when a guy needs it in the envelope. (William J. Gormley, Secretary-Treasurer of Teamster Local 470 in Philadelphia)

Mr. Gormley also pointed out that rapid increases in health care costs have caused the Teamsters Health and Welfare Fund in Philadelphia to run a $4.3 million deficit over the 1967 to 1975 period, resulting in a decrease in benefits such as the Teamster vision care plan. Other unions have also noted losses in benefits:

Lately we are being confronted with a major change by companies we have our contracts with—they are now taking the position that ... as increases in hospitalization costs take place they want our members to assume the cost .... We also have situations where in the case of benefits we already have in our contracts, the companies have indicated a strong move to remove some of those benefits in order to keep up with those rising costs. (Walter Kurkowski, Legislative Representative of District 7 of the United Steelworkers of America.)

The private sector is not alone in its inability to fund the present health care delivery system. For example, the Department of Health, Education, and Welfare (HEW) recently announced that it was required to increase the deductible for hospital coverage under Medicare from $124 to $144; the deductible was $40 when the program began in 1966.

These are all examples of the difficulty this society is having in meeting its aggregate health care bill and of an inability to commit more resources to health. However, it must be pointed out that inability to foot the health care bill may not mean that society needs to restrain health care spending. Inability to pay the bill may mean that too many resources are going to health. However, it is also conceivable that the allocation system lacks a capacity to provide the health field with the resources it deserves, given the prominence of health services as a social goal. For example, many conclude that this society's inability to fund the present health care system is evidence of a need for a national health insurance plan with very few controls on inflation.

Efficiency of Resource Utilization

Another concern is the efficiency with which health care resources are used. If the nation is to accept a tremendous rate of inflation in the price paid for health care, it must be persuaded that inefficiency does not exist. Unfortunately, even a cursory examination of the literature, including popular magazines and newspapers, reveals a list of misgivings about the efficiency of the present system:

1. The existing system with its several thousand independent units lacks effective coordination and planning, thereby leading to expensive and duplicative facilities, equipment, and services.
2. This uncoordinated system lacks comprehensiveness and continuity of care with the resultant possibility for duplication and fragmentation in the care provided to each patient.
3. Current financial arrangements for health care—fee-for-service or charges, and an emphasis on insurance coverage for inpatient care encourage consumers and providers to substitute expensive hospital services, which are insured, for uninsured and less expensive ambulatory care.
4. This financing system encourages providers to overprescribe or oversupply health services.
5. The present retrospective cost reimbursement formula for hospitals combined with the hospital's need to compete for physicians and the fact that a hospital's prestige is associated with the complexity of its case mix has led to the construction of expensive facilities and to the provision of highly complex services which are not fully used.[7]

A great deal of empirical evidence supports these criticisms. Open heart surgery and cardiac catheterization units are used so infrequently that the staff technical competence suffers, and wide observable variations exist in the amount of treatment provided for similar patients with little observable difference in outcome. There seems to be a wide concensus that health care does not use resources efficiently and that it is highly probable that the more resources committed to health, the more inefficiently those resources will be used.

Cost Versus Benefit

Analyzing whether the costs of health care are equal to the benefits is difficult for two reasons. First, the health care delivery system provides various benefits which are not directly related to health per se, and second, it is difficult to measure the impact that health care has on health status. For example, other benefits provided by the health care system include the employment of a great many people in an economy which presently has a high rate of unemployment, and some of the inflation in health costs is due to increases in employment and increases in wages within the health care industry. Health care also performs a "caring" function which may have little to do with health status but a great deal to do with human satisfaction.

Two major problems exist in measuring the impact of health care on health status: health in many respects is a self-defined state of being, and it is difficult to separate the effects of health care from the effects of other stimuli within the environment.

Given these problems in properly defining the shape of the cost-benefit equation, it appears possible to draw some conclusions about whether the costs of health care are equal to the benefits. Excluding for a moment the indirect benefits of health care noted above, there are several studies which have attempted to measure the impact of health care on health.

One technique used to measure this impact is to locate two populations with similar levels of income and access to medical care; Fuchs[8] compared the health status of the states of Utah and Nevada, and found the two states to be much alike in terms of income, schooling, degree of urbanization, climate, and other variables thought to be responsible for variations in mortality. Furthermore, the number of per capita physicians and the number of hospital beds are also similar. These are almost identical populations which devote similar amounts of resources to medical care, but the two populations rank at the opposite ends of the spectrum when it comes to health status as measured by death rates. (See Table 1-1) Since the amount of resources devoted to health care in these two states is essentially similar, what explains these wide variations in mortality rates? Fuchs concludes that "the answer most surely lies in the different life-styles of the residents of the two states. Utah is primarily inhabited by Mormons, whose influence is strong throughout the state. Devout Mormons do not use tobacco or alcohol and in general lead stable, quiet lives. Nevada, on the other hand, is a state with high rates of cigarette and alcohol consumption and very high indexes of marital and geographic instability. The contrast with Utah in these respects is quite extraordinary."[9]

Other studies arrive at similar conclusions. Auster et al.[10] examined the relationship between mortality rates and per capita medical expenditures across states, and concluded that there existed at best a small, statistically uncertain relationship. Another study conducted in England concluded that there was no consistent relationship between mortality rates and hospital admission rates.[11] Studies conducted in the United States have found that wide variations in utilization of health services cannot be explained by differences in risk factors or morbidity rates.[12]

Another approach to assessing the impact of health care is to measure improvements in health in a single population over a period of time as the amount of resources devoted to health care for that population is increased. One of the more widely known studies (McDermott et al.)[13] reports an attempt to improve health status on an Indian reservation by providing Indians with the best of modern medical care. Generally speaking, the researchers were not successful in improving health status relative to the amount of resources provided. Benham and Benham[14] looked at various populations with similar age and education levels, each of which had shown a large increase in hospital use. They found no correlation between self-reported health status, symptoms, and number of disability days and the increase in hospital use when other factors were held constant. Astvad et al.[15] studied the effect of increased use of resources on a specific health problem by analyzing the mortality rate from acute myocardial infarction before and after the establishment of a coronary care unit, and found no difference between the mortality experience of patients treated in the unit and those treated elsewhere.

Table 1-1

Excess of Death Rates in Nevada Compared
with Utah, Average for 1959-61 and 1966-68

Age Group	Males %	Females %
1	42	35
1-19	16	26
20-29	44	42
30-39	37	42
40-49	54	69
50-59	38	28
60-69	26	17
70-79	20	6

Source: Victor R. Fuchs, *Who Shall Live.* New York: Basic Books, 1974, p. 52. Reprinted with permission.

From this recounting of research results, it can be concluded that large observable variations in the amount of resources devoted to health care are not correlated with observable variations in health status. Devoting relatively more resources to health care, therefore, will not necessarily improve health status; conversely, devoting relatively fewer resources to health care will not necessarily harm health status. This does not mean that health care has no effect on health status. To the contrary, it is clear that basic health care, including prenatal and postnatal care, immunizations, treatment of infectious diseases borne by bacteria, and the setting of broken bones, improves health status. The problem illustrated by these studies is that present patterns of utilization indicate that society is far above the minimum level of health care which has significant impact on health. In economic terms, society has passed the point of diminishing marginal returns for health care, the point where the inputs of resources "exceed the point where the value of an additional increment to health is exactly equal to the cost of the inputs required to obtain that increment."[16]

Two additional points should be made. First, although society may be beyond the margin point in the aggregate, there are still portions of the population which are not receiving adequate health care and whose health status could conceivably be improved by more health care.[17] The second point is that health status could conceivably be improved by a different kind of health care. What the research does illustrate is that the present health care delivery system is doing just about all that it can be expected to do for health. Improved health status will have to come from somewhere else.

It is also necessary to return to the other benefits provided by the health care delivery system before this discussion can be concluded. Health is a labor-intensive industry providing many jobs at a time when the unemployment rate is high. If health care expenditures are reduced, or their rate of increase substantially slowed, jobs within the health care industry will be lost. In addition, health care provides a "caring" function which is not directly related to health. The question which must be asked is, are these two benefits or goals important enough to justify increasing expenditures for health in the absence of an improvement to health, the basic goal of a health care delivery system? The obvious answer is that this is a matter of social choice. The imperative of the health care delivery system, avoidance of negative impact on health, has been found not to be a problem when the resources devoted to health are reduced. This leaves society relatively free to decide whether increases in the resources devoted to health are justified by these other goals.

It is also necessary to ask if the "caring" function of health services are best answered by the highly technological style of care which the system presently produces in abundance. Perhaps those workers could better be used in a less expensive home-care system or in jobs designed to curb environmental hazards. It should be noted that 40 percent of health care costs go for hospital care, an area in which almost 50 percent of all costs are nonpersonnel costs. It can be suggested, therefore, that a cost containment policy which clearly recognizes the need to transfer personnel into less expensive settings, and which adequately recognizes the need to provide for needed "caring" functions, can contain costs without undue interference with these "other" benefits of the health care system.

Competing Goals

There is very little question that inflationary increases in the cost of funding the present health care delivery system are taking dollars away from the funding of other important social goals. Health expenditures accounted for 5 percent of the federal budget in 1965; they now account for over 10 percent.[18] This doubling of the proportion of the budget devoted to health has occurred during a period in which the total federal budget has more than quadrupled.

The list of other pressing needs to which part of the present health care budget could be applied is a long one. Furthermore, it is certainly conceivable, judging from the viewpoint provided by the research cited in the preceding section, that if society could find a way to relieve funds now allocated to health and apply them to some of the other pressing social needs, health status could be improved. Some of the other goals that come to mind are better housing, rebuilding the burned out Bronx, reducing safety hazards in the work place, removing carcinogens from the environment, improving schooling, and developing a nonpolluting and renewable source of energy. It is also true that in today's world society has a need to maintain a large defense establishment, although there is certainly a great deal of disagreement about how big it should be and how fast the nation should be moving to disassemble it. Nevertheless, it is interesting to note that the difference between President Ford's defense budget and former Secretary of Defense Schlesinger's proposed budget, was about $7 billion and their disagreement led to the secretary's resignation. For the same year, the relatively noncontroversial increase in the Medicare and Medicaid budget was over $5 billion.[19]

Inflation in the cost of financing the present health care delivery system also interferes with the funding of competing goals *within* the health care system. For example, complaints about the difficulty of finding a doctor or about crowded emergency rooms are common. Although the country has made great strides in equalizing utilization by the middle class and the poor since the introduction of Medicaid and Medicare,[20] reports are still published about pockets of the population that do not have access to care. Recent attention has focused on the poor rates of immunization among American children and the administration's new Child Health Assurance Program designed to deal with the problem.

Although these criticisms of the health care delivery system do not center primarily on costs, they do have a direct relationship. As long as health care inflation continues at a double-digit rate for essentially the same type of service, funds will more than likely not be available to make proposed improvements in the delivery of care. The secretary of Health, Education, and Welfare, Joseph A. Califano, Jr., expressed this point in his testimony on the Hospital Cost Containment bill:

> There are many serious health problems in this country—affecting rural citizens, the working poor, the aged and children—which simply cannot be met without diverting substantial resources away from costly and unnecessary hospital care. Attention to preventive and primary care, particularly for children, has suffered. Our proposed Child Health Assurance legislation is a good example of the need to redirect funds eaten up by hospital costs to improve essential services for low-income children. The voracious appetite of hospital charge increases can no longer be permitted to devour revenue needed for child health and other pressing health needs of the aged and the disabled.[21]

The secretary is an advocate for a particular piece of legislation, and cannot be accused of understating his case; nevertheless, an examination of the budget of the Department of Health, Education, and Welfare underlines his point. Between 1966 and 1978, HEW's annual budget for health increased 1,483 percent, from $3.0 billion to an estimated $44.5 billion. Of that increase, $37.3 was consumed by payments for Medicare and Medicaid, while only $4.2 billion was left over for expansion of other federal health programs beyond their 1966 level.[22]

Conclusions

The foregoing discussion on scarce resources and competing goals forms the philosophical base for this book. Clearly, not every person reading the analysis will agree with it. Some will point out, as was noted above, that society's difficulty in funding our present health care delivery system has nothing to do with the providers of health care services, but is simply a problem of financing mechanisms. They would say that rising health care expenditures are simply a matter of consumer preference and higher income and that distribution of funding is the problem, not the magnitude of those expenditures. In defense of their contention, they might note that when one looks at other countries with similar income levels, one finds that the proportion of the GNP devoted to health in the United States is not out of line.[23]

At the risk of being somewhat theoretical, a case can be made that these points are irrelevant. If a society decides that resources being committed to health could be used better elsewhere, it can choose to develop mechanisms to constrict the flow of resources to health. A problem exists, however, in reaching that decision, or, in more concrete terms, arriving at a political consensus strong enough to make such a firm decision.

It is not at all clear that this country has arrived at that consensus when it comes to health. President Carter has observed that "when Americans are asked, 'what in your life is important enough to raise taxes, if necessary?' the response is always, 'health care.' "[24] In addition, Herman Somers has pointed out that "there is no effective constituency in this country for cost containment (in health care). Therefore the prospects are not very good."[25]

This lack of support for the principle of constraint in health care costs appears odd when it seems to be so easy to point out examples of gross inefficiency in the use of resources in the health care sector. It is even more disturbing when one considers the lack of substantial evidence linking the provision of more health care with better health. Yet expenditures for health have been rising at a rate faster than the rise in the gross national product for over 30 years and, to date, there has been very little success in controlling that rise.

The Anatomy of
Health Care
Inflation

The purpose of this chapter is to provide a perspective on the how and why of health care inflation necessary to analyze the political actions taken to control it. The chapter displays the available statistical indicators associated with health care inflation in order to define clearly the problem with which the nation is attempting to deal. Trends in health care expenditures in terms of the proportion of total resources committed and the percentage increases in those commitments are discussed. Special attention is paid to the supply and use of resources in hospitals to illustrate the reasons for the present focus on controlling increases in expenditures for hospital care.

Trends in National Health Expenditures

National health expenditures amounted to an estimated $162.6 billion in 1977, a 12 percent increase over 1976. These expenditures, including public health services, administration, and research, in addition to personal health care expenditures, have tripled since 1965; they have multiplied more than tenfold since 1950. As well as increasing in the aggregate, national health expenditures have also increased dramatically on a per capita basis and as a percentage of the Gross National Product. Health care expenditures accounted for 4.5 percent of the GNP in 1950; 8.8 percent in 1977. Per capita spending for health care amounted to $78.35 in 1950 compared to $736.92 in 1977.[1] The trends in national health expenditures are shown in Table 2-1.

As Table 2-1 illustrates, total expenditures for health have been rising at a much faster rate than the rate of expansion in the economy. The 1977 GNP was about 18 times larger than that of 1929 while health care expenditures for 1977 were about 45 times larger. The rate of growth

Table 2-1

National Health Expenditures, Aggregate and Per Capita,
by Source of Funds and Percentage of Gross National Product,
Selected Years, 1929–1977

Year	Gross National Product (in billions)	Health Expenditures								
		Total			Private			Public		
		Amount (in millions)	Per capita	Percentage of GNP	Amount (in millions)	Per capita	Percentage of total expenditures	Amount (in millions)	Per capita	Percentage of total expenditures
Year Ending June										
1929	$101.3	$3,589	$29.16	3.5	$3,112	$25.28	86.7	$477	$3.88	13.3
1935	68.9	2,846	22.04	4.1	2,303	17.84	80.9	543	4.21	19.1
1940	95.4	3,883	28.98	4.1	3,101	23.14	79.9	782	5.84	20.1
1950	264.8	12,027	78.35	4.5	8,962	58.38	74.5	3,065	19.97	25.5
1955	381.0	17,330	103.76	4.5	12,909	77.29	74.5	4,421	26.47	25.5
1960	498.3	25,856	141.63	5.2	19,461	106.60	75.3	6,395	35.03	24.7
1965	658.0	38,892	197.75	5.9	29,357	149.27	75.5	9,535	48.48	24.5
1966	722.4	42,109	211.56	5.8	31,279	157.15	74.3	10,830	54.41	25.7
1967	773.5	47,897	237.93	6.2	32,026	159.15	66.9	15,853	78.78	33.1
1968	830.2	53,765	264.37	6.5	33,725	165.83	62.7	20,040	98.54	37.3
1969	904.2	60,617	295.20	6.7	37,680	183.50	62.2	22,937	111.70	37.8
1970	960.2	69,201	333.57	7.2	43,810	211.18	63.3	25,391	122.39	36.7
1971	1,019.8	77,162	368.25	7.6	48,387	230.92	62.7	28,775	137.32	33.3
1972	1,111.8	86,687	409.71	7.8	53,214	251.50	61.4	33,473	158.20	38.6
1973	1,238.6	95,383	447.31	7.7	58,715	275.35	61.6	36,668	171.96	38.4
1974	1,361.2	106,321	495.01	7.8	64,809	301.74	61.0	41,512	193.27	39.0
1975	1,454.5	123,716	571.21	8.5	71,348	329.42	57.7	52,368	241.79	42.3
1976²	1,625.4	141,013	645.76	8.7	80,831	370.16	57.3	60,182	275.60	42.7
Year Ending September										
1975	1,487.1	127,719	588.48	8.6	73,238	337.45	57.3	54,481	251.03	42.7
1976	1,667.4	145,102	663.06	8.7	83,560	381.84	57.6	61,542	281.22	42.4
1977²³	1,838.0	162,627	736.92	8.8	94,185	426.78	57.9	68,442	310.13	42.1

¹Revised
²Federal Fiscal Year
³Preliminary

Source: Robert M. Gibson and Charles F. Fisher. "National
Health Expenditures, Fiscal Year 1977." *Social Security
Bulletin*, 41 (July 1978): 3–30.

accelerated with the introduction of Medicare and Medicaid. In the decade before the introduction of Medicare and Medicaid, the average rate of growth was about 8 percent per year, while from 1966 to 1971, health care expenditures grew at about 12 percent per year. The period of the Economic Stabilization Program is the only period during which health care expenditures grew at a slower rate than that of the economy as a whole, even though health expenditures grew at an average rate of 10 percent per year during that period. Since that approach to cost containment expired, health care expenditures have been rising at an average annual rate of about 14 percent. This latest acceleration in the rate of increase occurred during the period in which the GNP growth rate has slowed appreciably. National health expenditures have also been taking an increasing percentage of personal income, rising from below 6 percent in 1950 to about 10 percent today.

The severity of the increases in national health expenditures is illustrated by comparing inflation in health to the inflation present in other sectors of the economy where it has been perceived to be a significant problem. An inspection of those rates shows that only energy-related prices have approached the rate of increase for hospital and physician services. The figures shown in Table 2-2 are from the Consumer Price Index (CPI) which is based upon the purchase prices for such specific items as prices for prescription drugs, semiprivate hospital room rate, and a physician's visit. To the extent that changes in these measures represent improvements in the quality of care, it is clear that the Consumer Price Index overstates price changes attributed solely to inflation. For the moment, though, it is sufficient to note that prices in the medical sector are inflating at a rate which is much more severe than the prices of other services. In fact, the controversy over how much the CPI misrepresents the relative importance of "pure" inflation and quality improvements is central to the political argument over the Hospital Cost Containment Act of 1977.

The Impact of Increased Health Expenditures

It is important to review the statistics which illustrate why increasing expenditures for health have become a political issue. The reasons for interest in the issue are fairly simple:

1. Public expenditures for health have been rising at a rate faster than health expenditures as a whole.
2. Expenditures by industry for employee health plans are, in many cases, the fastest rising cost of doing business.
3. Health expenditure inflation has direct impact on the cost of living.

Table 2-2

Comparative Rates of Price Increase:
1975, 1976, 1977

	Percentage Increase		
Consumer Price Index	1975	1976	1977
Consumer Price Index, All Items	9.1	5.7	6.5
Medical Care Services	12.6	10.0	9.9
Housing	10.8	6.2	7.0
Fuel, Oil, and Coal	9.6	6.6	13.0
Transportation	9.4	9.9	7.1
Apparel and Upkeep	4.5	3.7	4.5

Source: Bureau of Labor Statistics, 1977.

Public Expenditures. The public share of health expenditures grew from 13.3 percent in 1929 to 25 percent in 1950, a relatively modest rate, and then held at about 25 percent until 1965. After 1965, and the passage of Medicare and Medicaid, the public share has grown enormously, as shown in Table 2-3. The rapid inflation in public expenditures for health care is reflected in the increasing percentage of the federal budget devoted to health. Table 2-4 depicts the "health function" of the federal budget, which includes most federal health programs other than those in the Department of Defense and the Veterans Administration. If data for Defense and VA are included, health expenditures account for about 12 cents out of every federal dollar!

Expenditures for Employee Health Benefits. Expenditures for health benefit plans have risen substantially, both as a percentage of all wages and salaries and in absolute dollar terms. As was noted in the introduction, these increases are a cause of great concern for employer and employee alike. Employers have reported that since 1970 health insurance costs have tripled in some cases, while unions find that an increasing percentage of wage hikes are eaten up by health benefit increases. (See Table 2-5) These contributions for health benefits provide hospitalization benefits for 58 million workers, surgical benefits for 56 million, medical benefits for 55 million, and major medical benefits for 28 million workers. Although the number of workers covered for each type has grown, contributions have grown far more, as illustrated by Table 2-6.

Table 2–3

Public Share of National Health Expenditures,
Selected Fiscal Years, 1929–1977 (in Millions)

Fiscal Year	National Health Expenditures	Public Expenditures	Public Expenditures as a Percentage of Total
1929	$ 3,589	$ 477	13.3
1940	3,883	782	20.1
1950	12,027	3,065	25.5
1960	25,027	6,395	24.7
1965	38,892	9,535	24.5
1970	69,201	25,391	36.7
1975	123,716	52,368	42.3
1976	141,013	60,182	42.7
1977[1]	162,627	68,442	42.1

[1]Preliminary Estimate

Source: Adapted from Robert M. Gibson and Charles R. Fisher.
"National Health Expenditures, Fiscal Year 1977. *Social Security Bulletin,* 41 (July 1978): 3–20.

Impact on the Cost of Living. A rise in the costs of employee health benefits has indirect impact upon the consumer as the costs of goods and services must be increased in order to pay for those benefits. Increases in health care expenditures have direct impact upon the consumer through higher taxes and higher out-of-pocket costs for uninsured medical care. On the other hand, that there does not seem to be more public interest in this issue in light of the startling increases in expenditures for health makes it clear that the effects of much of this inflation are hidden from the public.

Trends in Hospital Expenditures, Prices, Costs, and Utilization

Thus far this discussion has illustrated the tremendous rise in total health care expenditures and its impact upon private and public expenditures to show the reasons why increases in health expenditures are an important problem and why these increases are receiving so much attention from health policy makers. It is important to note that most proposals for cost containment have been focused on the hospital sector

Table 2–4

Total Federal Outlays and Federal Health Outlays,
Fiscal Years 1966–1978 (in Millions)

Fiscal Year	Total Federal Outlays	Health Function Outlays	Health Function as a Percentage of Total Outlays
1966	$134,652	$ 2,638	2.0
1970	196,588	13,051	6.6
1975	326,105	27,647	8.5
1976	366,466	33,448	9.1
1977	417,417	39,505	9.5
1978[1]	459,375	44,485	9.7

[1]Projected Expenditure

Source: Office of Management and Budget, February 1977.

Table 2–5

Employer-Employee Contributions for Health Benefits
as a Percentage of All Wages and Salaries

Year	Health Benefits Contribution as a % of all Wages and Salaries
1950	0.61
1960	1.63
1965	2.15
1970	2.64
1971	2.80
1972	2.98
1973	3.02
1974	3.11

Source: Adapted from Alfred M. Skolnik, "Twenty-Five Years of
        Employee-Benefit Plans." *Social Security Bulletin,* 39
        (September 1976): 3–21.

of the health economy. There are several reasons for this, but the most important is that hospitals account for the largest share of expenditures for health and are second only to nursing home care in the rate of increase. That increases in hospital care expenditures have consistently outranked increases in other sectors of the health economy means that hospital care expenditures have been capturing an increasing portion of the health care dollar. As Table 2-7 illustrates, hospital care now accounts for over 40 percent of all health expenditures and has been increasing steadily for almost five decades.

Growth in expenditures made for any commodity in the economy is most simply explained by either a rise in the number of units purchased or by increases in the price of those units. Prices, in turn, are based upon the costs of producing those units, and, in classical economic theory, on the demand for those units and the available supply. In the hospital sector of the health economy, every one of the factors associated with increased expenditures has risen tremendously and each must be analyzed before it is possible to arrive at an understanding of why expenditures have risen so dramatically.

Table 2-6

Average Annual Increase in Covered Employees and
in Employer-Employee Contributions, 1950–1974.

Health Benefit	Average Annual Increase			
	1950–60	1960–65	1965–70	1970–74
Hospitalization				
Covered Employees	4.9	3.1	3.0	1.6
Contributions	16.1	11.6	11.8	10.9
Surgical—Regular Medical				
Covered Employees				
Surgical	7.8	3.0	3.5	2.2
Regular Medical	13.1	6.3	4.7	3.4
Contributions, Total	14.3	10.5	13.6	15.1
Major Medical				
Covered Employees	NA	13.5	8.2	3.5
Contributions	NA	18.1	16.5	18.9

Source: Adapted from Alfred M. Skolnik "Twenty-Five Years of Employee-Benefit Plans." *Social Security Bulletin,* 39 (September 1976): 3–21.

Table 2-7

National Health Expenditures by Type of Expenditure,
Amounts and Percentage Distribution,
Selected Fiscal Years, 1929–1977.

Fiscal Years	Total	Hospital Care	Physicians' Services	Dentists' Services	Drugs and Drug Sundries	Nursing Home Care	Other[1]	Research and Construction
				Aggregate Amounts (in Millions)				
1929	$ 3,589	$ 651	$ 944	$ 476	$ 601	$ NA	$ 650	$ 207
1940	3,863	969	946	402	621	28	763	134
1950	12,027	3,698	2,689	940	1,642	178	2,034	847
1960	25,856	8,499	5,580	1,944	3,591	480	4,068	1,694
1965	38,892	13,443	8,405	2,728	4,647	1,271	5,461	3,228
1970	69,201	25,879	13,443	4,473	7,114	3,818	9,338	5,137
1975	127,719	49,973	24,453	8,034	10,582	9,620	17,008	7,947
1976	145,102	57,497	28,504	8,519	11,472	10,834	19,073	8,734
1977	162,627	65,627	32,184	10,020	12,516	12,618	20,921	8,739
				Percentage Distribution				
1929	100.0	18.1	27.7	13.3	16.7	NA	18.1	5.8
1940	100.0	25.0	24.4	10.4	16.0	0.7	19.6	3.5
1950	100.0	30.7	22.4	7.8	13.7	1.5	16.9	7.0
1960	100.0	32.9	21.6	7.5	13.9	1.9	15.7	6.6
1965	100.0	33.8	21.6	7.0	11.9	3.3	14.0	8.3
1970	100.0	37.4	19.4	6.5	10.3	5.5	13.5	7.4
1975	100.0	39.1	19.3	6.3	8.3	5.5	13.3	6.1
1976	100.0	39.6	19.6	5.9	7.9	7.5	13.1	6.0
1977	100.0	40.4	19.8	6.2	7.7	7.8	12.9	5.4

Note: Rows may not add to totals due to rounding.
[1]Includes other professional services, eyeglasses and appliances, expenses for prepayment and administration, government public health activities, and other health services.

Source: Adapted from Robert M. Gibson and Charles R. Fisher, "National Health Expenditures, Fiscal Year 1977." *Social Security Bulletin*, 41 (July 1978): 3–20.

Utilization. Utilization is defined by two factors, the number of patients admitted and the length of time each patient stays in the hospital. Admissions to hospitals have risen continuously for the last 30 years. In 1946, there were 15,675,000 patients admitted; in 1977 there were over 37,000,000, a 235 percent increase over 1946.[2] Population growth was only about 40 percent during this period. In contrast, length of stay has decreased. Some of this decrease is explained by more frequent transfers of patients needing long-term care, especially psychiatric patients, to long-term care facilities or into ambulatory care programs. If one looks only at nonfederal short-term hospitals, length of stay has declined much more slowly, from 8.1 days in 1950 to 7.6 days in 1977.[3] Combining these figures, one finds that the number of patient days per thousand population has decreased for all hospitals, but has substantially increased for nonfederal, short-term hospitals. (See Table 2-8)

Costs. The most commonly used measures available for quantifying expenditures made by hospitals to provide care, developed by the American Hospital Association (AHA), are expense per patient day and per admission. AHA derives these figures by dividing total hospital expenses by the number of days of care or the number of admissions. These figures are then adjusted for the volume of outpatient care provided, thus arriving at a measure of expense per adjusted patient day and expense per adjusted admission. Table 2-9 summarizes the behavior of these measures since 1965.

Prices. Changes in the prices charged for medical and hospital care services are most commonly measured by the medical care components of the Consumer Price Index developed by the Bureau of Labor Statistics. As was noted above, because of the imprecision of the method in which a unit of service is defined, the CPI is insensitive to quality and intensity changes in the unit of service provided, but the index is useful to illustrate the inflation in hospital and medical care prices. Two CPI measures relate to hospital care. The first is the semiprivate room charge index, which measures charges for room, board, and routine nursing care in hospitals. In the early 1970s, the bureau developed a more refined measure, the hospital service charge index, which is a weighted average of separate charges for room, board, operating room, and eight specific services. As Table 2-10 illustrates, hospital charges have risen faster than prices in the rest of the economy except during the period of the Economic Stabilization Program. After the wage and price controls of ESP were lifted in 1974, hospital charges rose almost twice as fast as other services and, though the differential has eased somewhat, data for

Table 2–8

Inpatient Hospital Utilization in Non-Federal,
Short-Term General, and Other Special Hospitals,
Selected Years, 1950–1977

Year	Admissions (in thousands)	Average Length of Stay (in days)	Patient Days (per thousand population)
1950	16,663	8.1	879
1955	19,100	7.8	912
1960	22,970	7.6	966
1965	26,463	7.8	1058
1970	29,252	8.2	1163
1972	30,777	7.9	1145
1974	32,943	7.8	1188
1976	34,068	7.7	1194
1977	34,353	7.6	1182

Source: Adapted, with permission, from *Hospital Statistics,* published by the American Hospital Association, 1978 edition, © 1978.

the first nine months of 1977 show that hospital prices continue to rise somewhat faster than prices in the rest of the economy.

Supply. The supply of resources committed to hospital care has been rising just as dramatically as have utilization, costs, and prices. The number of beds per thousand persons staffed for use has increased over 25 percent since 1960. Employees per one thousand persons have increased over 70 percent in the same period while plant and equipment assets per thousand have tripled.[4] The number of hospitals which provide specialized ancillary services has also increased dramatically in the last 25 years. Tables 2–11 and 2–12 illustrate these trends.

The foregoing has provided a statistical portrait of the rises in hospital expenditures, the "how" of hospital inflation. As has been shown, every statistical indicator other than length of stay has exhibited a tremendous rise. The problem in designing a program to constrain these increases is to find the "why" of hospital inflation and then to design appropriate policies which will influence the factor or factors believed to be causing the inflation. The questions are numerous, and there is disagreement about which of many possible factors is the root cause of inflation in health care expenditures.

Table 2-9

Community Hospital Expenses per Adjusted Patient
Day and per Adjusted Admission, Selected Years,
1969–1977

Year	Expense Per Adjusted Patient Day	Annual Percentage Increase	Expense Per Adjusted Patient Admission	Annual Percentage Increase
1965	40.56	—	310.79	—
1966	43.66	7.6	337.54	8.6
1967	49.46	13.3	409.04	21.2
1968	55.80	12.8	471.30	15.2
1969	64.26	15.2	539.25	14.4
1970	73.73	14.7	610.10	13.1
1971	83.43	13.2	675.01	10.6
1972	94.87	13.7	749.47	11.0
1973	102.47	8.0	799.03	6.6
1974	113.55	10.8	885.69	10.8
1975	133.81	17.8	1026.79	16.3
1976	152.76	14.2	1168.78	13.4
1977	173.98	13.9	1324.27	13.3

Source: Adapted, with permission, from *Hospital Statistics,*
published by the American Hospital Association, various
years, © 1969–1978.

Table 2-10

Annual Rates of Increase in Consumer Price Index
and Selected Medical Care Components, Selected
Periods, 1960-1978

Consumer Price Index Components	FY 60-66	FY 66-71	8/71 to 4/74[1]	4/74 to 9/76[2]	1/77 to 9/77	8/77 to 8/78
CPI, all items	1.4	4.5	6.4	7.5	5.6	7.9
CPI, all services	2.2	6.0	5.1	8.9	6.4	8.4
Medical care, total	2.6	6.5	4.3	11.0	9.8	8.1
Medical care services	3.2	7.7	4.9	11.6	10.1	8.2
Hospital service charge	NA	NA	4.6[3]	13.4	11.2	NA[4]
Semiprivate room charge	6.0	14.6	5.7	15.4	11.9	10.8

[1]Economic Stabilization Program (ESP).
[2]Post-ESP controls.
[3]Annualized rate of change computed from January 1972, rather than August 1971.
[4]Measure discontinued December 1977. Its replacement "Hospital and and Other Medical Care Services," has increased 7.4 percent between December 1977 and August 1978.

Source: Bureau of Labor Statistics, 1978

Table 2-11

Trends in Number of Short-Term Hospital Beds and
Hospital Personnel, Selected Fiscal Years, 1950-1977.

Year	*Beds (in thousands)*	*Beds per 1,000 Population*	*Employees per Daily Census*
1950	505	3.3	1.78
1960	639	3.5	2.26
1965	741	3.8	2.46
1970	848	4.1	2.92
1975	947	4.4	3.39
1976	956	4.5	3.45
1977	974	4.5	3.60

Source: Adapted, with permission, from *Hospital Statistics,* published by the American Hospital Association, various editions, © 1950-1978.

Table 2–12

Trends in Hospital Facilities and Services,
Selected Years, 1950–1977 (Percentage of
Non-Federal, Short-Term Hospitals Having
Selected Facilities).

Facility	1950	1955	1960	1965	1970	1973	1977
Intensive Care Unit	NA[1]	NA	10.2	26.7	48.8	62.3	74.1
Intensive Cardiac Care Unit	NA	NA	NA	NA	42.1	35.0	35.3
Open-Heart Surgery Facility	NA	NA	NA	NA	7.1	8.5	10.0
Postoperative Recovery Room	NA	28.9	51.5	69.0	75.2	80.5	85.8
X-Ray Therapy	44.9	35.9	35.1	37.1	33.1	33.4	29.3
Radium Therapy	NA	NA	NA	32.0	27.5	26.5	22.4
Blood Bank	53.7	61.0	56.0	61.4	60.4	64.8	66.7
Electroencephalography	11.9	11.8	14.0	27.7	33.0	38.8	52.3
Inhalation Therapy Department	NA	NA	NA	NA	56.9	70.7	82.9
Renal Dialysis—Inpatient	NA	NA	NA	NA	10.3	11.7	15.2
Renal Dialysis—Outpatient	NA	NA	NA	NA	6.8	10.1	10.8

[1]Not available. The service was not included in AHA's survey at that time.

Source: *Hospital Statistics,* published by the American Hospital Association, 1977 edition, © 1977, reprinted with permission.

II | Theory and Practice

3 | Theories on Increases in Expenditures For Hospitals

There are essentially seven major theories which attempt to explain the rise in expenditures for hospitals, although there are variations on each and some are closely related to others. The following discussion provides an overview of the seven theories, with special attention paid to the role of third party payment and provider-induced demand as factors explaining rising hospital expenditures and costs. Although the conclusion reached assigns special importance to these two factors, it is important to note that each of the theories provides *some* explanation for hospital inflation, and the theories are very much interrelated. Categorizing them for purposes of discussion is, therefore, somewhat artificial.

Labor Cost-Push

Since hospital payroll expenses accounted for 50.3 percent of hospital expenditures in 1977, this component of hospital expense is a good place to start in any attempt to understand inflation in hospital costs. Labor expenses increased 13 percent in 1976 and 11.2 percent in 1977, a reflection of increases in the number of personnel as well as increases in wages.[1] Although increases in full-time equivalent personnel per inpatient day and per admission have been substantial, increases in wages have recently become a more important factor in payroll expense increase.

The labor cost-push theory of hospital inflation argues that tight labor markets, minimum wage laws, the growth of unionization, and a "catching up" process necessary to bring hospital wage schedules in line with the rest of the economy explain much of the inflation in hospital care expenditures. Table 3-1 compares the percentage impact of wage and price increases, and changes in labor and other inputs.

Table 3–1

Factors Affecting Increase in Community Hospital
Expense per Inpatient Day and per Admission,
Selected Periods, 1965–1976

| | *Average Annual Percentage Change* | | | | | |
| *Factor* | Expense/inpatient day[1] | | | Expense/admission[1] | | |
	1965–1971	1971–1974	1974–1976	1965–1971	1971–1974	1974–1976
Total Increase	13.0	10.2	15.2	13.3	8.6	15.1
Increase in wages and prices	6.7	5.9	9.5	6.7	5.8	9.5
Wages	8.1	6.0	9.4	8.1	6.0	9.4
Prices	4.1	5.5	9.0	4.1	5.5	9.0
Changes in Services	6.3	4.3	5.7	6.6	2.8	5.6
Labor	3.6	1.7	2.4	3.9	.2	2.3
Other	9.9	7.6	9.1	10.2	6.0	8.9
Percentage of increase due to:						
Wages and Prices	51.4	57.3	62.2	50.3	67.4	62.9
Changes in services	48.6	42.7	37.8	49.7	32.6	37.1

[1]Adjusted to exclude expenses for outpatient care.

Note: Price data are from Consumer Price Index, Bureau of Labor Statistics, all other data from Hospital Indicators, various years, American Hospital Association.

Note: Data for community hospitals includes units of institutions.

Source: Office of the Deputy Assistant Secretary for Planning and Evaluation/Health, U.S. Department of Health, Education and Welfare, 1977.

The underlying causes for the increases in wages are not clear and often contradictory. For example, Feldstein[2] has presented evidence that skill mix among hospital employees declined from 1940 to 1966, a situation which could reasonably be expected to have caused a decrease in wages. Davis and Foster[3] presented data to show a slight shift towards a higher skill level in hospital employees. There is little hard evidence in the literature to support the hypothesis that unionization is causing hospital wages to rise unreasonably compared to the rest of the economy, although papers by Lee[4] and Elkin[5] argue this point. In contrast, Bunker[6] found that wages rose slightly faster in nonunionized than unionized facilities in New York City during the 1960s.

The most pervasive theory concerning labor cost-push inflation is that hospital workers have been traditionally underpaid relative to other workers in the economy and are therefore going through a catching up process. Altman and Eichenholz[7] have pointed out that the increase in revenues available to hospitals with the growth of third party payers made it possible for wages to increase and for the differential between the wages of hospital employees and those in other industries to be reduced. The triennial Industry Wage Study in Hospitals conducted by the Bureau of Labor Statistics also demonstrates that a catching up process has occurred.

The problem with this theory as an explanation for today's inflation is that it would be expected that at some point equilibrium would be reached and inflationary pressure caused by wages would lessen. In fact, Feldstein[8] presented evidence that wages in some situations now exceed wages in comparable occupations. Evidence presented to the Subcommittee on Health and Scientific Research[9] of the U.S. Senate also substantiates this point. In other words, the catching up process is most likely over and, therefore, cannot explain either the sustained increase in hospital costs nor their magnitude.

There is some evidence in the literature that rising hospital wages may not be a root cause of inflation but are an effect of having unlimited revenue available to hospitals through the third party reimbursement system. Feldstein[10] hypothesized that hospitals may engage in philanthropic wage behavior by paying hospital employees more than would be minimally necessary to attract the necessary labor force. Since the third party system is thought essentially to insulate hospitals from any reduction in demand which might be caused by higher prices, it is to be expected that philanthropic wage behavior would lead to higher wages where a high level of third party payment provides substantially unlimited revenue to pay those higher wages. Through econometric analysis, Davis[11] has found that wages are significantly higher when patients pay a lower fraction of the bill out of pocket.

Regardless of the doubt cast upon the role of wage increases in explaining hospital inflation, most authors seem to agree that wage increases have played a substantial role. For example, McCarthy[12] notes that rising wages are an "undeniable fact," while Altman and Eichenholz[13] note that "although it is difficult to measure the precise impact of extension of minimum wage legislation to hospital employees, and the spread of collective bargaining agreements, there is little doubt that they have had major effects." Yet, even though the impact of higher wages has been substantial, as Davis[14] points out for 1966 to 1968, "the labor cost-push model of inflation does not provide a complete explanation of hospital inflation, since hospital costs per patient day would have increased at an annual rate of six percent even if wages had remained constant.'' Davis found that this rate of increase rose to 8 percent when she used data from 1966 to 1970.[15] Clearly then, because of doubt shed on wage inflation's role as a cause or an effect, and because of its lack of explanatory power, it is necessary to look elsewhere for the answer to the puzzle of rising hospital costs.

Lagging Productivity

Closely related to the labor cost-push theory is that increases in productivity in other industries push wage rates up. Hospitals must meet these higher wages to attract and keep an adequate labor force, but have limited ability to increase productivity themselves mainly because of their inability to substitute less costly capital for more costly labor.[16] There are several studies which have attempted to measure the impact of lagging productivity. A study by Lytton [17] compared productivity in eight federal agencies and only one, the Veterans Administration hospitals, exhibited no gains in productivity. Klarman[18] has stated that lagging productivity was the largest single explanatory factor of postwar hospital cost increases.

Unfortunately, a review of the literature provides a conflicting picture of the effects of lagging productivity. Feldstein[19] found a productivity decline of 3.8 percent per year using his method of constructing indices of real capital and labor inputs per patient day and then calculating the rate of change. In contrast, both Elnicki[20] and Cromwell[21] report productivity increases, although Cromwell reports increases for routine service departments and a decrease when both routine service and patient care departments are taken into account. Yet another study by Jeffers and Siebert[22] reports that gains in both labor and nonlabor factor productivity account for a reduction in the cost per case of 53.2 percent in three Connecticut hospitals over 10 years.

Regardless of the clarity of the research findings, the lagging productivity theory shares the same problem with the labor cost-push theory; it simply does not adequately explain the sustained inflation in hospital costs. Elnicki[23] points out that even if productivity gains could reach 9.4 percent, a rate six times higher than the most favorable rate found in the previously cited research, per diem costs would still rise 8 percent per year. Furthermore, increases in wages, no matter what the cause, cannot explain the inflation in hospital costs since costs would have increased substantially even if wage rates were held constant. [24]

General Cost-Push Inflation

In a paper on inflation in hospital costs, John McMahon, president of the American Hospital Association, and David Drake flatly state that "today's cost acceleration can be characterized as cost-push inflation. In other words, pressure stems from increases in the prices hospitals pay for resources needed to produce services and not from an increase in the quantity of services demanded."[25] AHA basically contends that the major reason hospital costs are inflating so much faster than prices in the rest of the economy is that the costs of goods and services which hospitals must buy (the hospital market basket) are inflating faster than general prices in the economy as reflected by the Consumer Price Index. AHA states that its own composite indices of hospital input prices suggests that prices in the hospital's market basket are nearly 50 percent higher than increases registered in the CPI.[26]

In testimony before the Subcommittee of Health of the Senate Committee on Human Resources, AHA asserted that its review of the approximately 15 percent annual increase in hospital costs indicated that "about ten percent of the increase is related to price inflation in the goods and services which hospitals must purchase to provide patient care, and the additional five percent is the result of increases in the intensity of services provided."[27] The evidence for this assertion is provided by the Hospital Cost Index (HCI) and the Hospital Intensity Index (HII) developed for AHA by Phillip, Jeffers, and Hai.[28] The HCI reflects increases in the price of 37 service elements used in the delivery of care to patients, while the HII tracks increases in the quantity of those same 37 services provided in a "typical" patient day. The behavior of these indices and of the CPI is illustrated in Table 3-2.

AHA argues that changes in the HCI are caused by forces outside of the hospital economy since the index is based upon the price of labor and nonlabor resources which are acquired by hospitals for producing the services used in the index, and because "each of the 37 services is defined as sharply as possible and the quantities are rigidly fixed."[29] In other words, the index is designed to avoid the problems of poor definition inherent in the CPI's use of vague terms such as "semiprivate room rate," for which the quality and intensity have clearly changed over the years. Instead the HCI uses much more specific terms, as illustrated in Table 3-3.

The problem with the index, as an inspection of the terms used reveals, is that it is not truly a measure of hospital input prices because increases in quality and intensity are still hidden within the terms used. AHA clearly admits that the HCI does not measure quality, but it is clear that their use of the term "quality" is synonymous with higher price. For example, the CPI uses the price of tetracycline as one of its index terms, a reasonably well-defined term. In the HCI, upward shifts in the unit price of "Pharmacy Line Items per Patient Day" could indicate a shift from the use of relatively inexpensive tetracycline to use of one of the exotic

Table 3–2

Movements of Consumer Price Index, Hospital Costs
Index, and Hospital Intensity Index, 1969–1976

Index	1969	1975	Average Annual % Increase 1969–75	Sept. 1976	% Increase 9/75 to 9/76
Consumer Price Index	109.8	161.2	7.8	172.6	5.5
Hospital Costs Index	100.0	153.3	8.9	171.1	9.0
Hospital Intensity Index	100.0	132.8	5.5	141.7	6.5

Source: P. Joseph Philip, "HCI-HII," *Hospital Financial Management* April 1977, pp. 20-26. Reprinted with permission.

Table 3–3

Sample of Terms Used in the Hospital Cost Index

Description	Quantity	Unit Price*	
		1969	1975
Clinical Laboratory Tests per Patient Day	2.35	$1.33	$1.51
Diag. Radiology Procedures per Patient Day	0.30	6.55	9.92
Nuclear Medicines Procedures per Patient Day	0.01	8.00	13.33
Pharmacy Line Items per Patient Day	0.96	2.27	2.24
Number of Meals Served per Patient Day	2.77	1.65	2.82
Pounds of Laundry Processed per Patient Day	12.91	0.07	0.11
Reg. Nurses Man-Hours per Patient Day	1.12	4.55	5.13
Med. Records Man-Hours per Patient Day	0.26	2.88	4.43
Adm. & Fiscal Man-Hours per Patient Day	1.33	4.52	7.83

*Unit price does not equal sales price. It is a measure of input prices.

Source: P. Joseph Philip, "Indices of Price and Intensity for the Hospital Industry," (Chicago: Hospital Research and Educational Trust, 1976) (processed). Reprinted with permission.

new antibiotics which tend to be much more expensive. Furthermore, use of the exotic antibiotics may not be as safe as the use of tetracycline, and using them could be termed a decrease in quality.

A true input price index would have to measure, for example, the price of a standard obstetrical pack of instruments or the price of a sheet of x-ray film. Using AHA's HCI index, there is the possibility that an upward shift represents an increase in the skill level of employees (for example, price increases in "Registered Nurse Man Hours per Patient Day" could be caused by hiring more master's degreed RNs) or by increases in the complexity of standard laboratory or nuclear medicine procedures. For these reasons one would have to view with skepticism AHA's assertion that pure inflation in the general economy is responsible for two-thirds of the inflation in hospital costs. Actually, the lack of a reliable measure of inflation in hospital input prices was one of the major concerns expressed by congressional committees in their deliberations on controlling hospital costs and led to amendments directing HEW to develop such a measure as quickly as possible.

A final point must be made about cost-push inflation. As noted above, some evidence has been presented to suggest that the extent of third party payment and wage rates levels may be interactive. It also certainly seems possible that increased third party payment may lead to increased nonlabor input prices. This would occur for two reasons. First, the substantially unlimited revenue provided by third party payment may mean that hospitals have little or no incentive to resist price increases in the products they buy. Second, hospitals have no incentive to purchase less expensive brands of similar products. For example, almost every major hospital supply firm carries a major brand's gauze products, and a house brand of its own. In many cases there is no difference in quality between the two brands, but the major brand frequently costs substantially more. The manager of one supply firm in San Francisco explained to the authors that only one hospital in that city, the county hospital with its high case load of medically indigent patients, buys much of the house brand while the other hospitals purchase the more expensive brand.[30] This is only anecdotal evidence, but cases of a manufacturer of lab equipment requiring the purchase of a certain very expensive solution as a condition of sale were brought to the attention of the Subcommittee of Health and the Environment during its review of cost containment in hospitals. Since it was found that cheaper solutions were available, it is reasonable to expect that if hospital management were more cost conscious, such practices would not continue. In sum, it appears that the role of cost-push inflation in hospital inflation requires a great deal more research. At present the evidence is uncertain, and there is little acceptance of the cost-push theory as an explanation of rising hospital costs. In fact, AHA appears to stand alone in its belief in this theory's accuracy.

The Relationship of the Labor Cost-Push, Lagging Productivity, and General Cost-Push Inflation Theories to Hospital Cost Containment Policies

The existence of these three theories is central to the congressional dilemma over hospital cost containment because, if one believes that these theories truly reflect the problem, controlling health care costs becomes much more difficult. If inflation in the health care industry is caused by factors outside the industry affecting prices for both labor and nonlabor inputs, then a logical way to cut hospital costs is to reduce services. Clearly, then, if one opposed the Hospital Cost Containment Act, it would be logical to persuade Congress that these theories explain much of the inflation in hospital costs, as the American Hospital Association tried to do in its testimony quoted above. The evidence which demonstrates that these theories only partially explain cost inflation should be extremely important in resolving this controversy.

Technological Improvements and Scientific Progress

The American Hospital Association's index of hospital intensity shows that the quantity of services provided to hospital patients has been rising at over 6 percent per year (see Table 3-2). Furthermore, intensity and "quality" increases may be even higher because of weaknesses in the AHA's measuring system. Another way of looking at the situation is to view the trends in payroll and nonpayroll expense per patient day as shown in Table 3-4.

As Table 3-4 illustrates, nonlabor inputs to care have increased in importance since the mid 1960s and this rise can be generally attributed to technological progress.[31] Technological improvements are thought to have impact on health care costs in several ways. Technology does not always provide a cure but, instead, provides a means to stay alive—a halfway cure—which involves continuing medical care. Renal dialysis is the best example of this since the end-stage renal disease patient never returns to full health and has a continual need for the renal dialysis machine.

Technological improvements appear to create their own imperative for use. This point can be understood by viewing the medical care system as being engaged in an unceasing battle against human disease. If one takes this view, and many physicians do, it can be seen that any weapon, no

Table 3–4

Trends in Payroll and Nonpayroll Expense per
Patient Day, Selected Years 1955–1977

| | *Average Annual Percentage Increase* | | |
Year	Total	Payroll	Nonpayroll
1955	8.2	10.0	5.6
1960	6.9	7.1	6.5
1965	6.7	6.4	7.0
1967	10.3	8.7	12.7
1969	13.8	12.9	15.1
1970	15.7	14.4	17.6
1971	13.9	13.7	14.2
1972	14.0	11.1	17.9
1973	9.0	6.8	11.9
1974	11.6	9.3	14.5
1975	18.3	15.1	22.1
1976	16.1	14.2	19.0
1977	14.2	12.5	16.5

Source: Adapted, with permission, from *Hospital Statistics,* published by the American Hospital Association, 1978 edition, © 1978.

matter how expensive, just might provide the cure or surcease from symptoms for which both the practitioner and the patient are striving. Most
physicians are not trained or equipped to conduct clinical trials, to
establish efficacy, or to analyze the costs and benefits. Furthermore, the
patient is apt to demand the use of a new procedure if it provides the one
in a thousand chance for survival. As McClure points out, "Why perform $50 of laboratory tests to be 95 percent sure of a diagnosis if $250
will provide 97 percent certainty? ... Or, if an annual physical is good,
why isn't a semiannual physical better?"[32]

There has been a significant rise in the provision of ancillary facilities
by community hospitals, and nonlabor inputs have increased faster than
labor inputs. Increases in nonlabor inputs have caused their share of
total hospital expenses to rise from 33.7 percent in 1960 to about 47
percent in 1977.[33]

One study widely quoted among congressional and HEW staff concerned with cost containment attempts to measure changes in the cost of
specific illnesses:

The average number of laboratory tests for perforated appendicitis increased from 5.3 per case in 1951 to 14.5 in 1964, to 31.0 in 1971. For maternity care, the number rose from 4.8 per case in 1961, to 11.5 in 1964, to 13.5 in 1971. Similarly, the number of x-rays per case of forearm fracture requiring a closed reduction with a general or regional anesthetic increased from 2.0 in 1961, to 5.4 in 1964, to 6.4 in 1971. For 1971, we estimated that the net additional inputs (compared to 1964 inputs) for appendicitis cost about $18.7 million in current dollars. Those with myocardial infarction cost about $275.2 million. Together these costs are about 0.4 percent of total personal health care expenditures in 1971. Considering that treatment in other conditions is likely to have changed in a similar way, the costs begin to mount.[34]

Other studies include one by Klarman[35] which found that ancillary service use accounted for one-fourth of the cost increases in the 1950s in New York. Two studies by Davis[36] found that for both the pre- and post-Medicare period, expenses for ancillary services exhibited a much higher rate of increase than did expenses for routine services. McCarthy[37] compared increases in plant assets to increases in beds and arrived at the conclusion that the square footage required to house sophisticated equipment is still rising.

Although this evidence suggests that technological improvement and scientific progress has a large impact on rising hospital expenditures, it does not explain precisely why this increase has taken place. For example, is the increase in the use of expensive technology explained by an increase in the elderly population, a population which spends about three times more per capita for health care than do those under age 64?[38] Preliminary analysis would reject this proposition because the percentage of the U.S. population over 64 has grown only from 8 percent to 10 percent over the last 25 years, while health expenditures have increased tenfold in the same period. In fact, both changes in the percentage of elderly and population growth are estimated to account for only about 10 percent of the total growth in health care expenditures.[39]

Nonetheless, medical advances have increased life span, and people of all ages who might have died earlier in life from poor pre- and postnatal care, or infectious diseases or other causes, now may very well live on to the point where they become victims of the chronic diseases which require more sophisticated and more expensive treatment. Increases in the complexity of the case mix faced by hospitals, therefore, would be a likely explanation of hospital cost increases as there are, for example, renal disease and heart disease patients being treated in hospitals today for whom no treatment was available in the past. However, the evidence on the impact of increases in the complexity of case mix on costs is not clear, although Davis[40] states that increases in the complexity of case mix can only explain about 7 percent of the overall cost increase. A definitive answer to this question will have to await the refinement and application of a methodology to assign resource use to case mix, as developed by Thompson and Fetter.[41]

There are, however, several points which suggest an answer to the question of the relative importance of technological and scientific progress in explaining hospital inflation. First, one would expect that if increases in the complexity of case mix were the answer needed to explain increasing hospital expenditures, the increased use of ancillary services would be mostly for the more complex, life-threatening diagnoses. In fact, Scitovsky and McCall[42] found that increased ancillary use was spread from the simplest procedures to the most complex; therefore, case mix complexity alone does not explain the tremendous increases in the use of ancillary services.

Much of the increase in ancillary service cost is caused by the use of services of dubious value or little cost effectiveness, and by duplication and inappropriate utilization of those services. For example, there have been no controlled clinical trials on coronary bypass surgery, a procedure costing from $7,000 to $10,000; further, there is evidence that for many bypass patients no benefit will be achieved and many others could have been treated as well with simpler, less expensive procedures.[43] The use of this procedure has been growing rapidly. Another example is gastric freezing for ulcer disease. This technique was widely adopted in the early 1960s without evidence as to its efficacy and against the recommendation of the American Gastroenterological Association.[44]

Extensive duplication in ancillary facilities is also reported throughout the literature. One example is the statement of Bernard R. Tresnowski of the Blue Cross Association before the Council on Wage and Price Stability: "Twenty out of thirty-two megavoltage radiation therapy installations failed to meet minimum use criteria established by a voluntary metropolitan health planning body for the 12-month period ending June 30, 1975. In that same area (Philadelphia), 16 hospitals have open-heart surgery programs, but only 5 used them enough to be considered efficient, to assure a desired level of quality."[45] The DeBakey Commission arrived at similar conclusions in the early 1960s, noting that 30 percent of the 770 hospitals with open-heart surgery facilities which were studied had no cases in the year under study.[46] Goldstein[47] found that certain sophisticated facilities which require a 70 percent occupancy rate to be cost effective actually have a 20 percent occupancy rate.

Although the existing research base makes it impossible to isolate the relative contributions of medical progress and of duplication to hospital inflation, it is certainly true that medical progress does not explain the existence of empty open-heart surgery units or the use of procedures of doubtful efficacy. This lack of explanatory power is made especially clear when one considers the results of several studies which have demonstrated that there is often little or no connection between increased use of exotic technology and good health. For example, the increased use of radiotherapy has had little effect on the age-adjusted mortality rate for breast cancer, while other studies have shown that coronary care units may not be effective and that many of those patients could have been treated just as well at home,[48] suggesting that a more complete explanation for inflation could be found elsewhere.

Several authors have attempted to explain the "technological imperative," noted above, and its impact on inflation. Aring[49] explains that physicians gain greater peer prestige from practicing high technology medicine than from practicing simpler, general primary medicine. Furthermore, physicians receive more income if they practice more specialized types of care.[50] It has also been noted that physicians are trained in medical centers where highly specialized, tertiary care is practiced, thus contributing to an acceptance of that type of practice as the norm.[51] Finally, the practice of "defensive medicine" has been noted by virtually every report on hospital costs issued in the last five years. Since malpractice awards have risen dramatically, there is a legal imperative to do everything that can possibly be done so that the physician can tell a court that an unexpected result is not due to omission. The effects of this practice are difficult to measure.

The incentives which lead to greater use of ancillary services by physicians directly influences hospital costs because hospitals must compete for doctors, and the hospital will be in a better position to attract physicians if it retains a full complement of services; "hospitals don't have patients; doctors have patients and hospitals have doctors."[52] A study by Rapoport[53] found that hospitals in competitive environments, areas with large numbers of hospitals, tend to acquire new technologies faster than other hospitals and purchase more expensive technologies. Pauly and Redisch,[54] Drakos,[55] and Buchanan and Lindsay[56] have also described the importance of physician incentives on hospital operation. Although each takes a somewhat different line, all three describe hospitals as a physician cooperative operated in the physicians' favor. The administrator's "own job security depends far more than on any other factor on his ability to keep the medical staff of his hospital satisfied."[57] One way to provide this satisfaction is to make available the latest medical technology.

Excess Capital Expenditures

A closely related theory of hospital inflation focuses on capital expenditures in general, although the theory draws on much the same data base as does the technological advancement theory. Proponents of this theory would point to the 400 percent increase in plant assets per daily census since 1950, and assert that this is the major factor in explaining cost increases.[58] The importance of capital investment in explaining hospital costs is underlined by the Department of Health, Education, and Welfare estimate that every dollar invested in a hospital capital asset will increase annual operating costs by $.50.[59]

One reason for growing capital expenditures is that the federal government has provided further incentives for capital expansion through funding of hospital construction. Between 1948 and 1971, nearly $13 billion was spent on hospital construction, nearly $9 billion for short-term hospitals; of the $13 billion, about 30 percent was provided by the Hill-Burton program.[60] Arising partially from this federal stimulus, the number of short-term hospital beds approximately doubled in the post–World War II period leading to a 33 percent increase in the bed-to-population ratio, from 3.3 beds to 4.4 beds per thousand persons.[61]

The issuance of tax-exempt bonds has become the major source of capital in recent years. Such bonds now account for 54 percent of all construction while direct government sources only accounted for about 3 percent.[62] Nevertheless, total capital expenditures are projected by HEW to reach $8.0 billion in fiscal 1978.

The result of this construction is that although patient days per thousand population in short-term care hospitals have increased, occupancy rates for those same hospitals have decreased about 2 percent since 1965 and presently stand at 74.4 percent for all nonfederal short-term care hospitals.[63] Underutilization, both in beds and in services, is especially important to costs because of the fixed/variable cost relationship. A lower occupancy requires allocation of a larger percentage of the fixed costs to each patient, thus forcing an increase in the per patient cost. Considering the evidence already presented concerning the amount of significantly underutilized specialized services, and the Institute of Medicine's estimate that there may be as many as 100,000 excess hospital beds in the United States,[64] the impact of uncontrolled capital expenditures on hospital costs is quite large.

Nevertheless, it is not clear whether capital expansion is a cause of hospital inflation or a symptom. The question arises because even though government provides financing or makes it possible for hospitals to issue tax-exempt bonds, the hospital must still generate revenue to pay

the operating costs of that capital facility, or to service the debt incurred
in building it. Hospitals seem to build these facilities without fear of any
losses, as evidenced by the low occupancy rates for services and facilities.
It seems not to bother the hospital industry that when one hospital builds
a cobalt unit or obtains a C.A.T. scanner across the street from another
hospital which already has those resources, both hospitals will have to
charge more for the service because of the resulting lower occupancy
rates.

It appears that hospitals engage in this behavior for several reasons.
First, it has been suggested that in addition to the desire of hospitals to
respond to the interests of the medical staff, there exist other important
incentives which motivate hospital administrators, boards of trustees,
and the community served by a hospital to expand the quantity of beds
and the quantity and complexity of equipment indefinitely. Size and the
complexity of services provided are the factors through which hospitals
compete and enhance their reputation.[65] Furthermore, as noted by
McClure:[66] "Powerful individuals—board members, donors, community leaders—for whom the hospital is a symbol and an avocation, can
easily become personally invested in these aspects. Additionally, administrators find building their hospital program personally rewarding, and
size can add financial stability if it can be financed. Hospital employees
want more secure jobs and employee unions want more jobs; both de-
sires are furthered by capacity expansion. The community tends to want
high quality services, all immediately available near home; it enjoys both
the prestige of its local hospitals and their economic impact on employment."

The second reason relates to third party payments which spread the
cost of expansion across many communities. As a result, no one
community has an incentive to reduce or prevent the powerful motivations which otherwise lead to expansion. Another way of looking at it is
that if one community decides to exercise restraint and all others do not,
that community will still pay for the expansionist trends of others even
though none of the benefits accrue to it. Similarly, the hospital has no
incentive to fight the provider's interest in a higher style of care and,
thereby, endanger its revenue base, since physicians will undoubtedly
transfer their patients to hospitals which do not curb expansionary
impulses. More importantly, widespread third party payment essentially
insulates hospitals from the effects of uneconomic decisions.

The Relationship of the Technological and Capital
Expansion Theories to Cost Containment

The significant base of evidence underpinning these theories provides a
solid basis for the belief that it is possible to control health care costs, at

least in the hospital segment of the industry. The evidence of unnecessarily complex styles of medical practice and of excessively expansionist capital investment suggests that restraints (or reductions) in the quantity of technological equipment, new services, and beds may be effected with little impact on health status. Moreover, the theories' suggestion that the key factor is the lack of resource constraints inherent in the third party payment system implies that decisions concerning the development of new services or more beds within a hospital might be made differently if some rational form of constraints could be imposed. The problem is that those resource constraints may not exist, as discussed in the following section.

Cost Reimbursement

This theory of hospital inflation asserts that it is precisely the lack of resource constraints under the present system of retrospective cost reimbursement which causes higher hospital costs. Essentially, this theory predicts that higher costs will occur because the reimbursement mechanism assures the hospital administrator that any increase in cost will be covered, as along as it falls under the definition of allowable cost. Because the establishment of Medicare caused the amount of medical care reimbursed at cost to increase 75 percent or more, evidence for this theory is mainly found in an analysis of pre- and post-Medicare costs. A good case can be made since the rate of increase in expense per day doubled after Medicare was established.[67]

On the other hand, studies have been unable to assert a direct relationship between cost reimbursement and inflation in hospital costs. As noted by Davis, "hospitals in states where cost reimbursement represented 88 percent of costs did not have higher costs, other things equal, than hospitals in states where cost reimbursement represented 19 percent of costs."[68] Davis also states that the percentage of cost reimbursed volume would have to reach 95 percent before the hospital would clearly have a cost raising incentive which could be ascribed to cost reimbursement alone.

Pauly and Drake[69] studied pre-Medicare costs in four states where Blue Cross employed different reimbursement methods. Their conclusions essentially parallel those of Davis. A study by Hellinger[70] indicates that hospitals manipulate their rate structure to maximize Medicare reimbursement through setting prices higher in departments with higher Medicare reimbursement. Although Medicare reimbursement is set by cost, higher prices would cause higher reimbursement because of the way cost is apportioned among departments. Hellinger's study may say less about the effects of cost reimbursement than about the hospital's desire to have a higher percentage of its total revenue provided by a steady, reliable source.

Regardless, the cost reimbursement theory as a single answer to the riddle of increasing hospital costs is difficult to accept since costs were rising significantly faster than the rate of inflation in the general economy long before Medicare was established. Just as in all of the theories presented thus far, cost reimbursement has most likely influenced hospital cost inflation but it cannot adequately explain it. As noted by Davis, "Medicare acted in much the same way as growth in private insurance to contribute to hospital inflation. This fact explains why the nature of hospital cost inflation was largely unchanged by the introduction of Medicare, although the extent of inflation increased dramatically."[71] This finding implies that the growth in insurance, i.e., third party payments, may be the important variable, regardless of which type of reimbursement is used. Canada with its universal health insurance has been experiencing cost escalation similar to the United States with its mix of private and public insurance.[72]

Demand-Pull Inflation and the Growth of Third Party Payments

As shown thus far, none of the theories displayed has sufficient power individually to explain all of the inflation in hospital costs. But there is another variable that has increased constantly over the entire period, the proportion of hospital costs paid by a third party, be it private or public insurance.

As illustrated by Table 3–5, the percentage of consumer out-of-pocket hospital care expenditures has fallen from 34.2 percent in 1950 to 5.9 percent in 1977. A basic statement of the theory explaining the importance of this variable is that increasing insurance costs provide an ever larger amount of revenue to hospitals with few resource constraints. The theory would further assert that insurance lowers the net out-of-pocket cost to the consumer, thus encouraging greater demand. There are, therefore, few resource constraints on the consumer who does not bear the burden of the entire price of hospital care, and there are few resource constraints on the hospital to avoid increases in the supply or complexity of that care since it is essentially free to pass on almost any cost to the third party payer.

The extent of health insurance coverage has grown tremendously over the last 40 years. The Health Insurance Institute of America[73] estimates that between 1940 and 1976, the number of persons covered by some form of private health insurance grew from about 12 million to over 171

Table 3-5

Amount and Percentage Distribution of Hospital Care
Expenditures by Source of Funds,
Selected Fiscal Years, 1950-1977

Fiscal Year	*Total*	*Direct Payments*	*Third Party Coverage*		
			Total	Private[1]	Public
		Aggregate Amount (in millions of dollars)			
1950	$ 3,698	$1,265	$ 2,433	$ 743	$ 1,690
1955	5,689	1,344	4,345	1,731	2,614
1960	8,449	1,583	6,586	3,348	3,508
1965	13,152	2,434	10,718	5,788	4,930
1970	25,879	3,174	22,705	9,553	13,152
1975	49,973	2,589	47,385	18,759	28,626
1976	57,497	3,423	54,074	22,046	32,028
1977[1]	65,627	3,866	61,761	25,561	36,199
		Percentage Distribution			
1950	100.0	34.2	65.8	20.1	45.7
1955	100.0	23.6	76.3	30.4	45.9
1960	100.0	18.6	81.4	39.4	42.0
1965	100.0	18.5	81.5	44.0	37.5
1970	100.0	12.3	87.7	36.9	50.8
1975	100.0	5.2	94.8	37.5	57.3
1976	100.0	6.0	94.0	38.3	55.7
1977[2]	100.0	5.9	94.1	38.9	55.2

[1]Includes private health insurance plus philanthropy and industrial inplant services.
[2]Preliminary estimates
Source: Adapted from Robert M. Gibson and Charles R. Fisher, "National Health Expenditures, Fiscal Year 1977." *Social Security Bulletin,* 41 (July 1978): 3-20.

million, while another recent study[74] estimates that over 94 percent of the population is covered by some form of public or private health insurance. Of this group, 71 percent are covered primarily through private health insurance policies, including Blue Cross/Blue Shield and health maintenance organizations; 10.5 percent primarily through Medicare; 7.4 percent primarily through Medicaid; and 4.9 percent through military programs, and Veterans Administration and other government coverage.[75]

A clue to the importance of this large increase in hospital insurance is found by comparing the percentage of hospital revenue provided by third party payment and the extent of hospital insurance, to the percentage of revenue and the extent of coverage for other services. This comparison reveals that while only about 6 percent of hospital revenue is from patients' out-of-pocket expenditures, about 35 percent of physician and about 85 percent of dentist revenue is from this source.[76] Similarly, more persons were insured for hospitalization, and more comprehensively, than for any other category.[77] Recognizing that hospital inflation is the most severe in the health care industry, the existence of greater protection from the usual resource constraints normally found in a market economy is especially significant. The research bears out this point. As noted by Davis: "The potential increase in hospital prices induced by insurance coverage is quite high. To illustrate this suppose that in the absence of hospitalization insurance a hospital could charge $100 per hospital stay and maintain a given level of capacity. A change to insurance coverage which reduces out-of-pocket costs to 20% of hospital charges permits the hospital to charge $500 per day without any increase in the out-of-pocket cost to the individual."[78] A leading proponent of this theory, Feldstein,[79] would argue that the situation described by Davis is precisely what has happened. Private income has risen while insurance coverage has caused net cost to the consumer for hospital care to rise much more slowly than income, thus leading to a greater demand for hospital care services. Hospitals raise prices without fear of losses in occupancy and use the larger revenue to raise wages, purchase more expensive equipment, and to invest in capital facilities. Feldstein studied state data on hospital costs for the period 1958 to 1967, and found that more than half of the rise in costs over that period was attributable to increases in private insurance coverage. A study of New York City hospital costs from 1961 to 1967 substantiates Feldstein's findings.[80] It attributed two-thirds of the cost increase to demand factors, defined primarily as increases in Medicare and private insurance coverage.

Davis has presented evidence in support of the demand-pull theory in several studies. One analysis, on the impact of Medicare, found that a 10 percent decline in out-of-pocket expense could be related to a 2 percent increase in average hospital costs, and further stated that: "There is no evidence to suggest claims that demand for amenities or added complexity of administrative tasks are primarily responsible for hospital inflation. Instead theories of hospital inflation that emphasize the role of specialized services, the expanded role of the community hospital, and advances in technology are all consistent with observed phenomena. The rapid increase in costs concomitant with the start of Medicare lends substantial credence to the view that hospitals respond to increased insurance coverage (either public or private) by changing the style (and expensiveness) of hospital care provided, particularly the areas of specialized services."[81] This point of view is especially significant since Dr. Karen Davis is one of the chief architects of the Hospital Cost Containment Act of 1977.

In another paper, Davis[82] asserts that demand variables (higher income and increased insurance coverages) account for 45 percent of the increase in hospital costs. Of special interest is that in reporting on the pre-Medicare period Davis finds significant increases in the factors which she later concludes are sensitive to demand-pull inflation: (1) an annual 3 percent increase in factor inputs; (2) a 52 percent increase from 1962 to 1966 in depreciation, interest, and rent expense, i.e., the costs of capital facilities; and (3) an increase in plant assets per day of 26 percent.[83]

Additional studies yield similar conclusions. Weisbrod and Fiesler[84] studied two Blue Cross subscriber populations, one of which had more comprehensive coverage than the other, and found that although admissions per thousand population decreased in both groups for the study year, admissions in the group with more comprehensive coverage decreased much less (13.8 percent in comparison with a 20.2 percent decrease in the group with less comprehensive coverage). The comprehensive group also received more ancillary services as well. Similarly, Feldstein[85] found that the proportion of the bill covered by insurance was a significant factor in the determination of hospital admissions, hospital days, and hospital expenditures, although he later failed to establish the significance of this variable in a study conducted with W.J. Carr.[86]

Rosenthal[87] conducted a study using state data for both 1950 and 1960, between which years the percentage of hospital revenue provided by private insurance almost doubled. He found that the percentage of hospital coverage was significant in explaining consumption of hospital services for 1960, but could not make this assertion for 1950 when insurance coverage was not as extensive.

Two studies using national data also indicate the importance of insurance coverage in predicting demand levels. Anderson and

Feldman[88] found that insured individuals use more of every kind of health service, while Andersen and Benham[89] found that extension of insurance benefits to low-income families caused a large increase in the demand for medical services.

Although these last six studies demonstrate the relationship between insurance coverage and increased demand, they do not necessarily show a relationship between the extent of third party payment and the ability of hospitals to increase the style, complexity, and expensiveness essentially at will, as suggested by Davis and Feldstein. In other words, the presence of more patients in the hospital does not necessarily suggest that the amount of services, employees, or capital assets *per patient* should have risen in such a dramatic manner. There are, however, several studies which begin to provide answers to this question.

Newhouse and Phelps[90] found that the choice of a hospital as measured by room and board charges is highly sensitive to coinsurance rates. Coinsurance is a form of resource constraint, and Newhouse and Phelps demonstrate that consumers will seek out a lower cost alternative if the costs affect them directly. Conversely, they will not if resource constraints do not exist.

Friedman[91] ties increases in insurance coverage directly to the increased use of resources by analyzing data from the Massachusetts Tumor Registry, and finds a doubling between 1965 and 1967 of the number of new cases of breast cancer treated by both surgery and radiation in this period in which Medicare was introduced. Breast cancer is one area in which mortality figures show little or no improvement.[92]

Two other studies suggest an important reason why hospital costs rise as the extent of insurance coverage increases. Joseph [93] related the extensiveness of third party payment to length of stay for 22 disease categories, and found that the relationship was significant for the 7 less serious conditions, indicating the importance of economic factors in the decision as to how much care is provided. Rosenthal[94] found that patients with more serious illnesses were less sensitive to net price variables than were the less seriously ill patients. These findings suggest that although increases in insurance coverage provide payment for health care which is vitally needed, it also provides payment for that which is not needed, i.e., the greater length of stay or those extra lab tests "just to make sure." It is also true that the hospital stay for most patients reflects a progression from acute illness to a state of better health at discharge. Thus it is possible to extrapolate from Joseph's and Rosenthal's research findings and point out that most patients would fall into the less serious category towards the end of their stay. It is, published research suggests, at this point that economic factors take over, and therefore it is possible to conclude that this situation occurs for many—and possibly—every patient.

These findings, then, provide a reasonably strong basis for acceptance of the demand-pull theory of hospital inflation. To reiterate, the theory states that increases in insurance coverage allow consumers to demand more services, thus providing more revenue to the hospital which is then able to use that revenue to provide more factor inputs. An important corollary of the theory is that the nature of the third party payment system, with its lack of effective constraints, allows health care providers to follow their powerful incentives toward providing a more complex style of care. Unfortunately, there is one flaw in this theory, and it is an important one. It is not the patient who decides whether or not to be admitted to the hospital; it is not the patient who decides that today there is a need for six times more laboratory tests than 20 years ago, and it is not the patient who decides the need for a computerized axial tomography scan instead of a simple skull x-ray. The consumer of medical care is generally as unaware of the possible diagnostic and treatment procedures which might be efficacious in dealing with an illness as one can possibly be. Regardless of statements from providers that demand has pushed up costs, it is clear that the articulation of that demand is not made by the consumer; it is made by the physician. This essential point is the basis for the last theory of hospital inflation to be presented.

Supply-Induced Demand

This theory builds upon the demand-pull theory and, in fact, changes it in only one way. Instead of stating that the consumer *demands* more care when third party coverage is extensive, this theory states that the consumer *accepts* more care when the coverage is extensive. Third party coverage, then, insures that providers will follow their powerful incentives to provide a more complex style of care and a larger quantity of that care than would be indicated by the relative health status of the population served. A kind of Parkinson's Law of medical care exists: "Standards of practice will eventually rise to absorb the dollars available."[95]

The importance of the provider in defining demand can be demonstrated by the percentage of the population which has seen a physician, the primary point of contact; this percentage is fairly constant across various populations.[96] However, there are large variations when one looks at more highly specialized care. The Social Security Administration[97] found that overall per capita admissions, patient days, length of stay, and expense show substantial differences even when insurance benefits are held constant. Wennberg et al.[98] studied small neighboring areas in Vermont and Maine and found that:

> Although there is an overall relationship between the rate of surgery and the number of surgeons, two areas with identical age-adjusted surgery rates achieved that rate by treating considerably different kinds of problems. For example, the area highest in overall procedures in 1969 ranked among the highest areas in tonsillectomies, hernias, and hemorrhoidectomies but among the lowest of the thirteen areas in appendectomies, chole-cystectomies, and hysterectomies. The area that ranked third in overall surgery was among the highest areas for appendectomies, chole-cystectomies, and hemorrhoidectomies but among the lowest for dilation and curettage and hysterectomies. Yet the evidence indicates that the distribution of health problems is the same among areas....The preferences of individual surgeons rather than differences in patient illness or access to physicians, we believe, are a more likely explanation for the variations in procedure rates.

Further evidence of seemingly random variation in procedure rates was related to a study of common surgical procedures conducted by Lewis.[99] The study found that across Kansas counties, these rates varied as much as twofold.

The important conclusion drawn from these findings is that the higher styles of medical care found by these studies are unneeded and, therefore, inefficient, since no correlation was identified between higher styles and better health. Information drawn from studies of health maintenance organizations (HMOs) provides further evidence on this point. Since HMO providers must attract and care for their enrollees within a total fixed budget determined by prepayment, which is in turn determined by market competition, providers within an HMO have an incentive to provide simpler, less expensive care. These studies indicate that after adjusting for age, sex, and other factors, HMOs use 30 to 50 percent fewer hospital days, fewer physicians, and provide health care at a cost 10 to 30 percent less than the traditional fee-for-service system. Moreover, there does not seem to be any measurable difference in health outcomes between HMOs and other styles of care.[100] The HMO evidence is particularly important in terms of cost containment because it indicates that when incentives are restructured, at least some providers will respond. Most significantly, the HMO evidence suggests that resource constraints can be built into the system without harming health status, assuming that those constraints will be constructed cautiously and carefully.

Perhaps a more basic point advanced by the supply-induced demand theory, and one with important implications for cost containment, is that the supply of health care resources may be the most important determinant of the demand for health care services. The first articulation of this argument was made by Roemer and Shain[101] with regard to hospital beds, and the principle which arose from their research is named after Roemer. Essentially, Roemer's law states that a higher bed supply independently predicts higher utilization. May's[102] statistical analysis found that a 1 percent increase in the bed supply would increase utilization about .4 or .5 percent.

Other studies take the argument a step further by linking physician supply and degree of specialization with patterns of hospitalization and the number and type of services. Feldstein[103] found that both per capita admission and mean stay per case are inversely related to the number of general practitioners but are positively related to an increase in the number of specialists and/or hospital beds, thereby demonstrating both the importance of physician preference and the independent effect of supply on demand. Studies by Nickerson[104] and by Hauck[105] further substantiate Feldstein's conclusion, observing that where there are more surgeons, a higher per capita surgery rate exists, although fewer procedures are performed by each surgeon. Fuchs and Kramer[106] have stated why supply is so important in explaining demand, suggesting that when physicians are plentiful, they may order services which are not medically indicated or are of marginal importance; when physicians are scarce, consumers may lower their expectations and deal with minor problems themselves. Although it suggests that a plentiful supply of physicians may increase utilization by lowering the nonmonetary costs of care (waiting time and travel costs), the study concludes that the physician's ability to control demand is most important in explaining higher utilization levels. A study by Evans[107] arrives at essentially the same conclusion.

Conclusions and Relationship of the Cost Reimbursement and Demand Theories to Cost Containment

The supply-induced demand theory does not stand apart from the other theories which have been presented; instead, it should be seen as building upon and further refining the other theories. It simply points out that it is the providers, both physicians and administrators, on whom various incentives, goals, rewards, and problems presented by the other theories have an impact. Furthermore, the theory implies that if the system can be restructured so that it has different impact on the providers, the other participants in the system (consumers, labor, auxiliaries, etc.) should be similarly affected.

This point can be highlighted by returning to the unanswered questions of each of the theories and noting their interrelationship with the lack of resource constraints contained within the third party system, and the ability of providers to induce demand. First, it was suggested that the three cost-push factors (labor costs, lagging productivity, and input costs) are effects of the third party system. The point was made that hospitals often pay more than they have to for both labor and nonlabor inputs, and this is most likely best explained by the ability of hospitals to increase their revenue without fear of a loss in demand for their services. By implication, restraints in hospitals' revenue-producing capability should lead to some reduction in inflationary pressure in these areas, although some inflation will doubtless continue in these costs.

Second, scientific and technological progress has contributed to care needed by a more elderly and more expensive mix of cases, although it was found that case mix and population variables account for a small portion of overall inflation. Science also has provided major advances in expensive technology which undoubtedly has driven up the costs of care. Unfortunately, alongside the beneficial advances in procedures and services, the use of services of dubious value or limited effectiveness without benefit of controlled clinical trials gives credence to the argument that many medical services are unneeded, and are inefficient producers of the ultimate goal—better health status. Furthermore, it was pointed out that the lack of resource constraints effectively circumvents any desire on the part of providers to engage in the cost-benefit analysis necessary to avoid this situation.

Not only does the third party payment system lead to use of inefficient resources, it also leads to the inefficient production of all those resources. It was pointed out that physicians have powerful incentives to demand highly complex and expensive services like the C.A.T. scanner, while hospital administrators have powerful incentives to provide those services. The present third party payment system insures that those services do not have to be used in an efficient manner, since the lack of resource constraints inherent in the system means that the hospital will be reimbursed for the service even though low utilization causes the price to be unreasonably high.

The evidence presented in this discussion has important implications for cost containment because it allows the strong assertion that costs can be contained through promoting efficiency in the use and production of hospital services without risk of a negative impact on health status. Placing constraints on the availability of resources would lead to a lessening of the tremendous duplication of services and facilities, and to a more critical posture in the evaluation of the choice of services to be provided.

Finally, the evidence suggests that the lack of resource constraints provides an inappropriately high level of resource utilization. Large variations in the number and type of services provided to essentially similar populations, and the independent correlation between the quantity of services available and their use, leads to the conclusion that constraints on the quantity of resources provided would lead to a lower level of utilization, and lower costs, again without risk of negative impact on health status.

The major variable which runs through all of the theories, then, is that the hospital care system lacks the resource constraints normally found in a market economy, while containing many incentives which lead to an ever increasing use of resources. The evidence presented suggests that if some type of resource constraint could be imposed, behavior would change and the rate of inflation would be reduced.

A point to keep in mind, however, is that this evidence only *suggests* that resource constraints can favorably affect costs without unfavorably affecting health. It does not specifically indicate the desired changes in behavior, nor does it definitively answer the question of what level of resources should be provided. It is fairly easy to say that waste exists at the macroeconomic level; it is a far more difficult task to decide what, in fact, is wasteful at the microeconomic level. For example, it is not at all clear which of the higher number of tests provided to appendicitis patients are definitely needed and which are not. Moreover, the structure of the present third party payment system precludes the need for gathering that information. Therefore, any proposed cost containment system will most likely have to be imposed in an incremental fashion—a slow tightening process—and the statistical indicators of health status, patient mix, complexity of services, and financial viability of health care providers will have to be closely monitored throughout the process.

In proceeding to a discussion on past and present actions and proposals designed to constrain the rate of increase in resource use in health care, it is especially important to keep in mind the importance and high regard for health care accepted by this society. Because of this high regard, the burden of proof is on those who would curtail the resources going to health, not the physicians and hospital administrators who consume those resources. For this reason, control mechanisms must be carefully designed and proven operationally, so that the public and their representatives are convinced that efforts to control costs are not hindering the production of needed health care services. In consideration of the difficulty in defining the proper level of resource use, this task is not an easy one.

4 | Previous Governmental Efforts to Contain Hospital Costs

Previous governmental control efforts fall loosely into three general classifications: (1) controls on reimbursement; (2) controls on the supply of facilities and services; and (3) controls on utilization. Each type of effort discussed has provided important experience, or is seen as an integral part of the present effort to control hospital costs, the Hospital Cost Containment Act.

Reimbursement: The Economic Stabilization Program

The most extensive effort to control the level of hospital reimbursement was the Economic Stabilization Program (ESP) lasting from August 1971 to April 1974. During this period, ESP was relatively successful in halting the hospital cost spiral as hospital inflation was reduced below the inflation in economy-wide prices. Unfortunately, as soon as the program ended, rates of increase in hospital expenditures rocketed upward once again. Clearly, the program had few long-term effects on inflation in the health care industry, and its failure to do so provides important evidence on how controls might be structured.

ESP began with a 90-day freeze on wages and prices in the entire economy (Phase I). Phase II consisted of more specific controls for each major sector of the economy, although controls on different industries were similar. HEW had argued that the health care industry "had sufficiently unique problems and business practices" to allow it to be controlled separately, but was unsuccessful in this argument.[1] This caused immediate problems since, under the unique hospital reimbursement system, it was not clear whether the controls applied to charges or to cost-based payments made by third party payers. This problem was clarified through regulation by defining cost-based payments as "prices" for purposes of controls.[2]

The next problem was whether controls were to be applied to prices per unit of service, prices per day, or prices per admission, and this situation was not clarified until regulations were released nine months after Phase II started. The regulations stated that increases in aggregate annual revenue due to price were limited to 6 percent, with the following limitations on increases due to costs: (1) aggregate wage and salary increases were limited to 5.5 percent; (2) aggregate nonwage and nonsalary current expenditure increases were limited to 2.5 percent; (3) aggregate increases for new technology and new services were limited to 1.7 percent.[3] There was also considerable ambiguity concerning the base to which these limitations would be applied, and how the effects of volume increases or decreases would be measured. This issue was resolved in July 1972 by deciding that the controls would apply to "the amount of [the hospital's] aggregate annual revenues for its most recently completed fiscal year (adjusted for volume differences)."[4] Finally, in recognition of the upward trend in inputs per patient day, a 2 percent intensity factor was added bringing the total allowable increase up to 8 percent.

One problem with the program became immediately obvious: the ambiguity of the regulations, and the several attempts to clarify them, made it difficult for hospital administrators to comply with the directives. Furthermore, the program more than likely removed any incentives to comply since it was almost impossible to know if one was in compliance at any point in time.[5] Another problem involved the volume index which did not differentiate between marginal and average costs. Research by Feldstein[6] and Lave and Lave[7] demonstrates that hospital marginal costs tend to be lower than average costs, thus causing the cost per admission to decrease as the number of admissions rise and to increase as admissions fall. Instead of recognizing these differences in the rate of change associated with increases and decreases, ESP's volume index simply raised or lowered reimbursement by an amount equal to the average cost of each admission gained or lost. In effect, this rewarded hospitals with increasing volume and penalized those with volume decreases, clearly inappropriate for a cost containment program. In fact, there was an unusually high increase in admissions during this period.[8]

It has also been pointed out that the program's assumption that hospital nonlabor cost increases would be held to only 2.5 percent was overly optimistic. Although ESP attempted to hold economy-wide price increases to that figure, many hospitals found that they could meet the 5.5 percent labor cost limitation but not the 2.5 percent nonlabor limitation.[9] This led to a reclassification of expenditures to those which could qualify under the 1.7 percent allowable increases in new technology and services.

The arbitrary nature of the 2.5 percent limitation on nonlabor input increases also led to a high volume of exceptions. This unexpected large volume of requests for exceptions led to establishing state advisory boards to rule on these requests. The test used was elementary; those institutions experiencing a negative cash flow, and which were found by the state advisory board to be needed for the health care of the community, would be granted an exception. Since the test of "need" was almost invariably met, the net effect of the exceptions process was to remove any incentive to control costs, since the hospital could simply push up its costs to the point where it was in danger of experiencing a negative cash flow, and then request an exception.

An additional problem experienced during ESP was that the base period data on which all of the calculations were made came from the hospital's own data, a problem which still exists today. This meant that many hospitals were not limited by the controls.[10]

In sum, the Economic Stabilization Program had mixed success. Hospital expenditures as a percentage of gross national product remained fairly steady during its life and the rate of increase in hospital service charges dropped by half. On the other hand, it contained within itself incentives to raise costs and volume and to increase technological inputs. It is interesting to note that although price increases dropped 50 percent, cost per patient day and per admission dropped only about 25 percent, leading one to assume that cost-based payers were subsidizing charge-based payers during this period.[11] This finding, plus the fact that all statistical indicators resumed their inflationary spiral as soon as the program ended, makes it clear that the program had little effect in changing the structure of the hospital economy. It is of particular interest to note that the rate of increase in total hospital assets *rose* from 11 percent in 1971 to 13.5 percent in 1972, and remained above 11 percent for the duration of the program.[12] In other words, regardless of the imposition of controls on revenue, hospitals continued to find funds to finance the expansion of capacity, which has been found to have such an important impact upon total hospital expenditures.

Given the problems of Phase II, and the Phase III extension of its controls, the Cost of Living Council drew up new control regulations for the health care industry which were implemented as Phase IV on July 1, 1973, following the economy-wide freeze which had begun on June 13. Although the new program contained many innovative features which might have alleviated the problems noted under Phases II and III, the new program was aborted when controls ended on April 30, 1974. Therefore, it had little opportunity to influence behavior in the health care industry. Many of the Phase IV control features, however, are contained in the Hospital Cost Containment Act of 1977; this may result from the fact that many of the same HEW hospital reimbursement specialists who were involved significantly in the design of the ESP Phase IV guidelines also helped draft the 1977 cost containment proposal.

Included in the Phase IV guidelines was a change in emphasis from per diem expenditures to per admission expenditures, thereby removing any incentive to increase volume by increasing length of stay or by increasing volume of ancillary services. The guidelines also attempted to reduce the incentives towards increased admissions by specifically taking marginal costs into account. Under Phase IV, hospitals which experienced a reduction in admissions of 5 percent or less (10 percent in the case of small hospitals) would have suffered no loss in allowable revenue. Beyond this point, allowable revenue would have been reduced by only 40 percent of the allowable per admission amount. This adjustment would continue until the hospital reached the point at which allowable per admission revenue for the remaining admissions had increased by 20 percent. Similarly, hospitals with increasing admissions received no increase in revenue for a 2 percent increase, and only 40 percent of the allowable per admission revenue for increases higher than that, except that a further adjustment was provided for hospitals with a very large increase (9 percent for large, 12 percent for small hospitals).[13] Both the emphasis on per admission cost and charges, and the volume (or fixed/variable cost) adjustment are included in a somewhat different form in the Hospital Cost Containment Act of 1977.

One of the major questions left unanswered by ESP is which level of government should control the mechanisms designed to alleviate hospital inflation. The program suffered from many methodological problems, and its most sophisticated effort was terminated before it could have much impact on hospital economy; it is, therefore, difficult to use the experience of ESP as a benchmark for the likely success or failure of a federal program like the Hospital Cost Containment Act. It is important to point out, however, that two of the major architects of ESP, Stuart Altman and Joseph Eichenholz,[14] have concluded that:

> The experience of the Economic Stabilization Program showed that the kinds of sensitivity required in a prospective reimbursement system makes it impossible to administer it equitably at the federal level for very long. Phase II contained many specific examples of inequity and hardship suffered by hospitals—each of whom had to be handled as an exception. The Phase IV system recognized the limitations of the federal government effectively to administer a system of strict controls, and would have allowed a qualified state authority to administer any or all aspects of a cost-control program that seemed consistent with ESP goals. It was and still is

the feeling at the federal level that a state-level group is able to administer any prospective reimbursement system more equitably than is the federal government.

Within this statement is an implied challenge to state governments to take the initiative in hospital cost containment. Furthermore, the federal government has supported the development of state cost containment programs through funding authorized under the Social Security Amendments of 1967 and 1972, and Section 1526 of the National Health Planning and Resources Development Act of 1974. The following section highlights the efforts of those state programs which are commonly thought to be the most advanced in the field.

State Cost Containment Programs

Presently nine states (Colorado, Connecticut, Maryland, Massachusetts, New Jersey, New York, Rhode Island, Washington and Wisconsin) have mandatory state cost containment programs in operation.[15] Six other states have enacted cost containment programs which do not mandate compliance with the program's directives; in at least ten others, voluntary programs are operated by state hospital associations or by Blue Cross. Thirteen additional states reportedly are considering action in the cost containment area.[16]

All of the mandatory programs use some form of prospective reimbursement, although there are great differences among the actual methods used to implement this general principle. Simply put, prospective reimbursement involves a system which sets a level of payment for services in advance which is applied to a specific period of time in the future. Essentially, prospective reimbursement is a form of resource constraint intended to curb the excesses found under the present retrospective reimbursement system, i.e., inefficient use of resources, low occupancy, maintenance of excess capacity, and provision of services of limited value. It may be seen that the success of prospective reimbursement systems in effecting these changes in health system behavior depends on how tightly the prospective reimbursement system is drawn, for clearly a prospective system which allows for a high rate of increase will not be successful in altering behavior. In contrast, a system which provides too little revenue may be detrimental to *needed* health care or the quality of the care provided. The problem is to design a system which is sensitive enough to take into account the myriad differences among different institutions (teaching versus nonteaching, rural versus urban, small versus large, etc.), and to structure the system such that incentives built into the program do in fact alter behavior in the direction desired.

A variety of prospective reimbursement systems have been designed, implemented, and evaluated. They fall into three general groups: (1) budget review approaches which involve a detailed review of institutional budgets upon which is based either approval or setting of rates, or the setting of a total allowable revenue amount; (2) formula methods which involve the use of inflation formulas to set ceiling or target rates; and (3) negotiated rates which involve the hospital and the rate setter in a joint decision-making process.[17]

The problem of setting a reasonable level of reimbursement when the variation among hospitals is so large has been dealt with in various ways. Maryland uses a detailed budget review which attempts to verify the true costs of any service and then aligns the cost with the service. The hospitals whose rates for a particular service fall in the top 20 percent of all hospitals are then challenged. Washington State uses a peer review system in which hospitals are grouped on 18 variables and each group is then screened for higher values. Both systems arrive at a prospectively approved budget through use of these methods and through negotiation. The major point which can be drawn from observing these systems is that they both use a detailed, sophisticated methodology designed to be as sensitive as possible to the special needs and circumstances of different institutions.

Another interesting concept which is being implemented at the state level is the attempt by New Jersey to tie reimbursement directly to the case mix of a hospital, although the effort is in its very early stages. This system would measure the resources consumed by each type of patient as determined by the patient's diagnosis. Then patients would be divided into diagnostic review groups.[18] A prospectively approved rate would be set for each diagnostic review group as determined by the resources consumed by that group, and the hospital's reimbursement would be determined by multiplying that amount times the number of patients within each group which the hospital served. The total amount would then be adjusted for changes in volume, quality, or inflation.[19]

An important question is deciding on the base to which the prospective reimbursement system should apply. Various programs use prospective hospital reimbursement on a per diem, per admission, and rate per specific service basis, and each contains its own set of incentives. Dowling[20] pointed out that a per diem basis encourages hospitals to monitor the cost per day, but also encourages it to increase the number of patient days. Evaluations conducted by the Office of Research and Statistics of early experiments in prospective reimbursement in six states found that the number of days increased under the per diem system.[21] Similar incentives operated under per admission and per unit of service systems, with both leading to a higher volume of services. The programs thought to be the most successful (Maryland, Connecticut, and Washington) all have moved toward a system which sets a total allowable revenue budget with some adjustment for volume.

Volume adjustments, though, are also a difficult problem. The problem is to identify the marginal (or variable) cost of a unit of service. As in the ESP program, volume adjustments which provide for a one-for-one increase, or decrease, in revenue as volume increases, or decreases, contain an incentive toward increasing volume. If a hospital gains (or loses) only the marginal costs associated with an increase (or decrease) in volume, there is a smaller incentive toward volume increases, and a positive incentive toward volume decreases. This occurs because the revenue *per admission* will increase as volume decreases, as only the marginal cost of the reduction is subtracted from total revenue. The most sophisticated example of this type of adjustment is used in Washington where different marginal cost assumptions are applied to different sized hospitals, an assumption which appears to fit the actual situation more closely.[22]

Although several states have instituted imaginative cost containment programs, the evidence on their success or failure is open to question. As noted by Stephen Weiner, chairman of the Massachusetts rate-setting commission, "The state of the art of rate setting is fairly primitive."[23] There are many problems yet to be solved. For example, the evaluation conducted by the Office of Research and Statistics reported that early systems effected only a 1 to 3 percent savings over the retrospective reimbursement system, and the evaluators further noted an increase in volume in many of the programs.[24] However, these findings have been held to be significant because they represent the first careful documentation to indicate that prospective reimbursement affects hospital costs.[25]

McCarthy[26] noted that some programs have relied upon the possible rewards under a prospective reimbursement system (those hospitals containing costs at a level below the prospectively approved level can earn a "profit") and concluded that the small rewards possible are insufficient to counteract the incentives now present which drive costs up. The problem which results is that penalties must then be used to achieve modification of the system, and those penalties must be drawn so that hospitals which provide needed care are not driven into bankruptcy or into inappropriate reductions in the quality of needed care.

Worthington[27] has related an additional problem suffered by some cost containment methods: the chosen system actually reinforces existing inflationary trends. This occurs because the prospective rate was established on the basis of the previous year's actual costs, thus providing an incentive to spend as much as possible in one year as a means of receiving a higher level of revenue the following year. This problem can be avoided by using peer review, as in Washington, or by using triannual line-by-line budget review based upon normative costs, as in Maryland, rather than on historical trends used in the New Jersey system studied by Worthington.

Regardless of the problems noted by these authors in the operation of the earlier cost containment methods, the newer systems in Washington, Maryland, Massachusetts, and Connecticut are beginning to show significant results. According to HEW,[28] preliminary estimates for 1977 indicate that the national rate equalled 14.2 percent with Connecticut at 11.4 percent, Maryland at 11.8 percent, and Massachusetts at 13.7 percent. Although the Washington program was not operative until the middle of 1977, the state's preliminary findings indicate that an increase of only 4.6 percent per patient day and 5.8 percent per admission will be allowed in 1978. This would translate into an increase in net revenue of 11 percent.[29] It is especially interesting that in at least two states the rate setters are beginning to change behavior in the industry to the extent that constraints on revenue are starting to cause hospitals to make decisions which lower their costs. This is evidenced in Maryland by an improvement of the financial conditions of hospitals from a deficit position when the rate-setting commission began operation to a current profitability factor of 1.14 percent.[30] Washington's rate-setting commission reports: "Preliminary studies indicate that the overall financial position of hospitals in Washington has improved slightly, despite the significant reductions in the rate of increase in costs to patients. The implications of these preliminary studies are that hospitals are applying more stringent management controls, improving their efficiency and productivity, yet without the sacrifice of their overall financial position or the quality of care provided to patients."[31]

Unfortunately, the results achieved by these programs have not been formally evaluated. Nonetheless, it is important to note that the Health Insurance Association of America[32] has supported the establishment of state rate-setting commissions. Perhaps even more significant is that the American Hospital Association[33] passed a resolution to its House of Delegates meeting in Washington, D.C. in February 1978 putting that organization on record in support of state rate and budget review.

The existence of such support from these organizations provides evidence of the strengths of state cost containment programs. First, state programs have generally used a process which is selective enough to deal with individual circumstances, a factor which has earned the grudging support of hospital associations in the states involved. Second, they have controlled costs sufficiently to persuade the insurance companies that their financial position will be improved by the rate setters' actions. Third, each state has been able to experiment with various control methodologies. This point is especially important in consideration of the "primitive" state of the art of hospital reimbursement controls.

The major problem in fostering the development of these types of programs is that it is not at all clear that the experience of Washington, Connecticut, Maryland, Massachusetts, New Jersey, and a few others can be translated to every state. Each of these states benefits from talented people who have been the driving forces behind the rate-setting commissions. Of concern is what happens when rate setting becomes a traditional and routine function of state government, rather than the new and different experiment that it is now. There is also a pervasive fear that hospital regulators may follow the route of regulators in other industries and will begin to serve the interests of the regulated rather than of the public. Both of these questions certainly bear careful evaluation, as does the general question of the success or failure of state programs in containing hospital costs.

Even if the programs prove to be successful in limiting hospital revenue, it is not clear that they would be successful in limiting total expenditures for hospital care since, except in Connecticut, rate-setting commissions can have impact only indirectly on the rate of growth in the supply of facilities and services in hospitals. This responsibility is lodged in another type of public agency.

Supply

The major statutory authority for attempts to constrain the rate of increase in the supply of hospital services is contained in the National Health Planning and Resources Development Act of 1974, and in Section 1122 of the Social Security Act. Under the Planning Act, 205 regional Health Systems Agencies (HSAs) are required to review and recommend to a State Health Planning and Development Agency (SHPDA) whether proposed hospital capital expenditures over a specified amount or changes in hospital services are needed by the community. The SHPDA then must review the proposal and the recommendation, and grant a certificate of need only to those services and facilities for which a positive finding of need has been made.

The concept of certificate of need, however, did not originate with the 1974 national health planning law. The first statutory certificate of need program was enacted in New York State in 1964 and, although provisions vary widely, by early 1979, 41 states had enacted legislation. The first federal recognition of certificate of need occurred in the Social Security Amendments of 1972 in which Section 1122 required the secretary of HEW to enter into agreements with states which were willing and able to review the need for proposed hospital capital expenditures. Under the 1122 program, HEW withholds depreciation and other costs related to an expenditure found to be unneeded when reimbursing health care facilities for services provided under the Medicare, Medicaid, and Maternal and Child Health programs. Thirty-three states review capital expenditures under the 1122 program.

As a result of Section 1122 and individual state action, all but one state (Missouri) review hospital capital expenditures, although there are wide differences in the methods used to conduct reviews. The 1974 Health Planning Act is significant in this regard because, for the first time at a national level, it requires all states to have a certificate of need program which is satisfactory to HEW and, through regulations promulgated on January 21 and April 8, 1977, it has established consistent minimum requirements for a satisfactory program. The law further provides that any state without a satisfactory program by the end of fiscal year 1980 cannot receive any federal funding under the Public Health Service Act and other related health authorities until a satisfactory program is in operation. It is also important to note that the 1974 law also requires HSAs and SHPDAs to work actively toward shaping the health care delivery system in their respective areas of responsibility through the development of Health System Plans and Annual Implementation Plans, as well as through reviewing the "appropriateness" of health facilities in their areas at least every five years.

Considering that certificate of need is the major cost containment strategy available to planning agencies, it is important to analyze how successful it has been in constraining the increase in the supply of facilities and services. Unfortunately, contrary to the hopes of many health care policy makers, the program does not appear to have enjoyed much success thus far. Empirical analysis of the five earliest programs shows that between 1968 and 1972 existing programs reduced growth in the number of hospital beds by only about 9 percent; however, in consideration of the independent effect the supply of beds has on hospital utilization, the analysis shows that utilization averaged about 4.8 percent below what could have been expected in the absence of a certificate of need program.[34]

These early results were updated to 1974, a period during which the number of certificate of need programs increased to 25. Unfortunately, the analysis found that no decrease in the rate of growth in beds occurred in the 20 states with new programs, while plant assets per bed and total assets in those states actually increased beyond the level expected without a certificate of need program. The evidence on the five early programs was somewhat better as analysis indicated that expenditures per capita, taking into account both capital costs and utilization, were somewhat lower than expected in the absence of a certificate of need program; the maximum decrease amounted to 3.1 percent.[35]

In defense of the health planning agencies, it has been pointed out that these regulatory efforts are in their infancy, and that there has been little in the way of standards and criteria needed to guide the agencies in their deliberations. The difficulty of the health planner's job is underscored by noting that in the period reported in the above study (1971 to 1974), total plant assets in hospitals grew by 40 percent.[36] The planners are essentially trying to induce cutbacks in an industry that has tremendous incentive toward expansion. Without defined standards and criteria, it is difficult, if not impossible, to say no to those who would expand. The result is that 92 percent of all projects reviewed were approved by the ten state level health planning agencies investigated by the General Accounting Office in 1976.[37]

Problems in the timely development of standards and criteria for review highlights one of the major issues in implementing the Planning Act. In September 1977, HEW released a Notice of Proposed Rule-making which contained ten standards "respecting the appropriate supply . . . of health resources" as required by the Act.[38] These standards provided that there should be no more than four beds per thousand population in any health service area, and an occupancy rate of at least 80 percent. There were also supply and occupancy standards respecting obstetrical beds, neonatal intensive care units, pediatric beds, coronary units, C.A.T. scanners, radiation therapy units, and end-stage renal disease units.

Although the department called the guidelines a "major step forward in our efforts to control rising health care costs and to assure quality health care for the American people," the furor began immediately.[39] HEW received over 50,000 separate pieces of mail in opposition to the guidelines, mainly because it was mistakenly assumed that the guidelines gave HEW the right to close hospitals or services. This misunderstanding was mirrored in Congress, as evidenced by the following statement which Paul Rogers, chairman of the Subcommittee on Health and the Environment (which has jurisdiction in the House of Representatives over the Planning Act), felt compelled to make:

> The primary misunderstanding is that the guidelines will be used to force hospitals, particularly hospitals in rural areas, to close. *There is nothing in the health planning act that requires or authorizes* the Health Systems

Agency, the State Health Planning and Development Agency, or *HEW to close hospitals,* services, or facilities. The application of the guidelines may *identify* unneeded facilities in an area, but changes in existing services must be brought about *voluntarily* as the law is currently written. [Emphasis added.][40]

The prevailing view on the guidelines was stated by Mr. Kazen of Texas:

I cannot imagine any agency of this government trying to hold hearings on guidelines that propose to close or curtail services being performed by certain rural hospitals, but also a lot of metropolitan hospitals because of some silly guideline that they not be within 45 minutes reach of another facility.[41]

Perhaps the major criticism leveled against the content of the guidelines was that they were "cost control" guidelines rather than guidelines designed to improve access and quality, although it is not clear why cost control guidelines are not proper when costs are escalating at the present high rate. Regardless, the effect of the outcry was that HEW revised the proposed guidelines to make it clear that HSAs and State Health Planning and Development Agencies could deviate from the guidelines if they found that using them would cause substantial disruptions in access to needed health care services. Moreover, in their 1978 proposals to extend the Planning Act, both the House and Senate committees removed the requirement that health plans be "consistent with" the guidelines, which further weakened their impact. The only possible conclusion is that very few people have accepted the argument advanced in Chapter 3 that substantial reductions in capacity could be achieved without a negative impact upon the quality of health care or upon health status.

Although health planning has not been particularly effective in containing health care costs, the argument over the guidelines and the recent hearings held in Congress on extension of health planning authorities have demonstrated that there is high interest in the program. It appears that the health plan development, certificate of need, and appropriateness review functions of the health planning agencies contain the tools to begin reallocating health care resources in a more efficient fashion if those tools were used aggressively, notwithstanding the present opposition to the close-out of excess capacity. It is interesting to note that New York State has had some success in closing out excess capacity, although this has been achieved by holding reimbursement rates to a level low enough to force hospitals into bankruptcy. Similarly, an imaginative program in Detroit has attempted to identify some of the steps which must be taken if excess capacity is to be reduced, most important of which is actively to seek public support before any action is taken to close hospital facilities.[42] It appears that health planning will enjoy greater success as the dimensions of the cost containment problem become more widely known, and persons outside of the health care system begin to take a more active interest in doing something about it. The increasing participation of many business executives in the health planning process is evidence that this is already occurring.[43]

An interesting bit of anecdotal evidence of the increased awareness concerning health planning is that the efforts of one HSA to preclude a hospital from building a $5 million, 84-bed addition were recently described in Sylvia Porter's lay-oriented column, "Your Money's Worth." The column points out that although the HSA did not approve the hospital's application, the state overruled the HSA, thereby allowing the hospital to build the facility. Unfortunately for the hospital, Blue Cross cancelled its contract due to noncompliance with the HSA's decision. Porter concluded, "Learn about and honestly participate in local health planning activities. . . . If a hospital or hospital expansion is needed, support it. If it is not needed, oppose and stop it. If you act, you can contribute to curbing your own health-care costs. If you do not act, your failure will result in all of us paying more and more for health care, directly or indirectly—as taxpayers, patients, health insurance subscribers, and employers."[44]

Regardless of the success or failure of health planning, responsibility for the other major component of health care costs, utilization, is lodged in yet another effort, the Professional Standards Review Organizations (PSROs) mandated by P.L. 92–603. For although ratesetters may design systems which provide incentives against inappropriate utilization, and health planners may constrict the number of facilities and services, these actions have impact only directly upon utilization. If utilization continues to rise, or if a high degree of inappropriate utilization exists, costs will remain unnecessarily high, regardless of the reasonableness of the charge for the services or the efficiency of the institution in which the service is provided.

Utilization

Professional Standards Review Organizations are private regional bodies operated by local physicians and charged with the review of the appropriateness of institutional utilization of Medicare and Medicaid patients. The PSRO effort contains three major components: concurrent review, medical care evaluation, and profile analysis. Concurrent review, through preadmission certification and continued stay review is designed to insure that hospital admission and continued stay are necessary, with the goal being a reduction in the number of units of care purchased per individual. Medical care evaluation is intended to encourage study of problem areas and to develop corrective action. Profile analysis is defined as "the presentation of aggregated data in formats which display patterns of health-care services over a defined period of time."[45] Particular analysis of diagnosis-specific, institutional, practitioner, and patient profiles is mandated.

The PSROs are almost as new as the HSAs and have suffered from some of the same kinds of organizational and definitional problems. Although the program is very young, there is a great deal of skepticism about the ability of the program to control costs, mainly because of concern about the willingness of physicians to police themselves. In fact, the Office of Management and Budget recommended to the president that PSRO funds be deleted from HEW's fiscal 1979 budget, and it took a strong appeal on the part of Secretary Califano to have the funds included.[46] Part of the problem is that the American Medical Association maintains that the program is not a cost containment program, but rather a quality assurance program, and that the review process should be used to eliminate poor medical practices rather than to reduce admissions or length of stay.[47] This point was brought out in the 1977 HEW evaluation of the PSRO program which noted: "Professional Standards Review Organizations have become different things to different people. In the DHEW implementation of the program, the quality assurance aspects of the program were emphasized in order to gain the cooperation of physicians. On the other hand, the literature associated with the history of the legislation in Congress perceived a cost-containment orientation. This has tended to produce differing sets of views throughout the health care community regarding the program's objectives."[48]

Because of the youth of the PSRO program, there is little hard evidence available on its success or failure in containing costs. What evidence does exist provides few examples of success in curbing unnecessary utilization of services of federally sponsored patients. This may result from the poor role definition extant in the program, or because administration of the program was divided into two HEW divisions before the Health Care Financing Administration was created in 1977.

The most exhaustive study of the PSRO program to date is the 1977 HEW Office of Planning, Evaluation, and Legislation (OPEL) study quoted above. The OPEL study found no aggregate PSRO effect on the utilization variables studied, although it was found that some *individual*

PSROs were associated with lower utilization. In comparing the effects of PSRO review on Medicare and Medicaid utilization, OPEL found smaller decreases in case mix–adjusted average length of stay for Medicaid patients in hospitals under PSRO review than in non-PSRO hospitals, and greater decreases in length of stay for Medicare patients. However, the study reports that PSRO review is associated with increases in severity of case mix for Medicaid patients, thus allowing the tentative finding that PSRO review may be causing bed days to be used more efficiently for Medicaid patients. The most negative finding contained in the OPEL study, and one which may have led to the Office of Management and Budget's recommendation to President Carter to terminate PSRO funding, was that in order to pay for itself through offsetting reduced utilization in the federal reimbursement programs, the PSRO program would have to reduce utilization rates of covered groups by 1.6 to 2.05 percent. As OPEL noted, "study findings imply that, even though certain PSROs have demonstrated this degree of cost-effectiveness, the PSRO program is not now cost-effective and thus is not yet serving as a cost-containment mechanism."[49] Nevertheless, OPEL cautioned against reaching final conclusions about the program since the study had been conducted during a time when the program was in its developmental stage.

Other studies of PSROs and PSRO-like organizations have provided similar inconclusive, and at times inconsistent, evidence about the program. Studies in Utah[50] and New Mexico[51] found little or no evidence of reduction in admissions or length of stay. Research on the effects of programs in Colorado and California, however, found significant reductions in utilization rates, but results are questionable because neither study controlled for trends in reduced utilization before the advent of the PSROs.[52] Although clarification of the inconsistent evidence must await further research, a clue to the problem is contained in the structure of the PSRO. Most PSRO review activities are delegated to individual hospital review committees, and in studying three hospitals the Institute of Medicine[53] found that significant savings were present in only one. Moreover, this hospital engaged in aggressive planning for patient discharge, thus providing patients and their physicians with alternatives to inpatient care. The OPEL study also found that greater reductions in average length of stay were evident in PSRO areas with higher supplies of long-term beds.[54]

As in the health planning program, the PSROs are charged with combatting some of the incentives which exist now in the hospital care system. Clearly, it will take aggressive management and creative design if the PSROs are going to have an impact upon utilization. It is also just as clear that as long as all other incentives in the system are directed toward higher utilization, the physicians who are expected to carry out the mandate of the PSRO program will not have any particularly good reasons for implementing that mandate, especially as it relates to reductions in utilization. It has been pointed out that preadmission certification would provide the best possibility for reducing utilization. Not surprisingly, the PSROs are generally not involved in such an activity.[55]

Conclusions

The Economic Stabilization Program provided some evidence that health care costs can be contained, but the program was instituted in the context of economy-wide wage and price controls and the impact is unclear. The furor over the National Health Planning Guidelines and the continuing controversy over the proposed Hospital Cost Containment Act emphasize that control of health care costs is a difficult political and social task. In an industry whose product is widely accepted as necessary, if not crucial, to the well-being of the public, and in which the real costs are hidden through a third party payment system, any effort to constrict the flow of resources to that industry will undoubtedly engender serious opposition. Further, with the tremendous problems of defining what is needed, and what is a reasonable level of reimbursement, not to mention Americans' general opposition to centralized planning and control, it is possible to conclude that no sweeping, centralized control methodologies will have much chance of success. Regardless of the lack of progress evidenced by the three localized control methods described above (state rate review, health planning, and the PSROs) the one thing in their favor is that they involve local citizens in the design of solutions to rising health care costs and, therefore, may earn the support of those citizens for whatever control methodologies are ultimately used. It may be a very slow process, but it also may be the only strategy possible in this field.

Another important theoretical strength of the three regionally based efforts is that each is charged with the collection of data about the health care system, and these efforts should provide the kind of information necessary to make decisions about resource use in health care. Moreover, the universe to which these efforts are being applied is small enough that the information should be specific and adequate to identify where resource use is too high and where it is too low. In consideration of the problems faced by cost containment efforts (insuring that only unneeded facilities are closed, that individual hospital budgets represent efficient and "reasonable" use of resources, and that the care provided is needed by the community), the importance of collecting these data cannot be overemphasized.

In fact, much of the difficulty of analyzing the impact of the Economic Stabilization Program, and the 1977 Hospital Cost Containment Act, is caused by the lack of specific data. Individuals opposed to the cost containment effort often cite the deleterious effects of ESP, while those in favor claim just the opposite. It appears true that ESP reduced the rate of increase, and it is also true that ESP had no measurable impact on the indicators of health status including the age-adjusted mortality rate, the infant mortality rate, age-adjusted death rates for selected causes, and age-adjusted life expectancy.[56] This lack of impact on health status may be explained by ESP's short-lived effect, and the ability of hospitals to absorb short-term losses and to defer costs. The ratio of current assets to current liabilities in hospitals decreased considerably during the period of ESP, according to the American Hospital Association.[57] Nevertheless, in line with the theoretical conclusions predicted in the literature, ESP should have had an impact on hospital decisions on utilization, expenditures, and expansion. Unfortunately, the data to show this impact are either unavailable or aggregated on too gross a level; therefore, it is difficult to use ESP as a model or guide to implement the 1977 cost containment legislation. In the best of all possible worlds, the data collection efforts of the HSAs, PSROs, and state rate and budget review agencies would have been in place during ESP, and specific national data thus made available on the effect of revenue controls.

Also to be pointed out is that the lack of specific information on individual hospital revenues and expenditures, marginal and average costs, utilization, and expansion imposes restrictions on how tightly a national program can apply resource limits. This problem may be avoided by regional and state planning and regulation agencies, given their abilities to experiment with different methods. If the states find that a method is ineffective, too expensive to administer, unworkable, or has a negative impact on health care services determined necessary, it can be modified or scrapped fairly easily; most state rate review programs have gone through a succession of different budget methodologies. The ability to experiment also means that regional programs can begin implementing a control program relative quickly, without waiting for the definitive methodology to be finely tuned.

Regional programs, which collect specific data on the shape of the health care system in their area, have another important theoretical ability not included in a program like ESP; they directly influence many of the factors which contribute to rising costs. For example, an HSA and a state health planning agency can prevent the construction of excess resource capacity; a PSRO can discern and apply constraints to unnecessary utilization; and a state rate or budget review agency can conduct a comparative budget review which identifies those institutions operating in an inefficient manner. In comparison, ESP applied gross wage and price controls which were expected to force hospital administrators and physicians to take a more critical stance toward introduction of new capacity, higher utilization (except when controls were on a per diem basis), or inefficient management.

Finally, through coordination of their efforts, regional programs having direct impact upon the cost-increasing factors within the system theoretically can deal with the inherent conflict of interests which invariably occurs when resource constraints are applied. In the case of budget review and health planning, the conflict occurs because planners are concerned primarily with question of need and access while budget reviewers focus primarily on costs. In a time of limited health resources, the overall goal must be to identify the best need/access/cost trade-off. Budget reviewers might interfere with the resolution of need and access problems by putting inappropriate constraints on the revenue necessary to operate needed institutions. On the other hand, planning decisions taken in the absence of cost criteria may perpetuate the status quo and, therefore, continue the tremendous inflation now present in the health care system.

Underutilized services lead to further problems in the absence of coordination, as many of the cost inefficiencies which budget reviewers attempt to eliminate are caused by underutilization. When a service is underutilized, unit cost is high because of the need to spread fixed costs over a smaller number of patients. If budget review commissions attempt to lower the allowable operating costs for such a service, questions of community need and access undoubtedly will result. This problem could be avoided if health planners provided the budget review commission with recommendations associated with an assessment of need. Also, planning recommendations might be employed by budget reviewers to use the reimbursement system as a means of encouraging the production of services required to meet outstanding community needs or to discourage, or phase out over time, the production of unneeded or duplicative services.

Utilization review and quality assurance efforts conflict with planning and budget review activities. A budget review system which focuses on restricting unit costs may produce incentives which result in an increase in both the quantity of resources and volume of utilization. The PSROs are required to produce data on utilization which, if provided to the budget reviewers, might contribute to the disallowance of excess revenue produced. Similarly, the possibility exists that a hospital with an inappropriately high utilization rate might be granted a certificate of need by the health planners on the basis of the apparent demand, thereby being rewarded for inappropriate practices in that institution. Utilization profiles could help to avoid that situation.

The major concern of the PSROs, quality assurance, may also be impaired by the efforts of budget reviewers and planners. There is an operational difficulty in measuring quality in an objective sense, but it is possible to use existing process measures to obtain a general picture of the quality of care provided in an institution. Results of medical audit and utilization review data could be coordinated with hospital cost profiles to provide an assessment of the quality of care provided in an institution relative to its costs.

These activities, however, are the theoretical possibilities for health planning, state budget and rate review, and utilization review and quality assurance. Many of the basic activities of these efforts have not been implemented on a widespread basis; coordination is especially weak.[58] The present proposal for containing costs, the Hospital Cost Containment Act of 1977, is based partially on the idea that national limits must be imposed within which these regional efforts can be carried out. It is argued that without a national program, regional efforts will continue to be ineffectual. For this reason, the Hospital Cost Containment Act has direct impact on local planning, budget review, and quality assurance efforts, and much of the argument surrounding the legislation is concerned with identifying the proper role of regional activities in a national cost containment program. The lack of hard evidence on the success or failure of the regional programs has crucial import in the deliberations over whether the new cost containment proposal is needed. Moreover, the local character of the planning, budget review, and quality assurance programs, and their *theoretical* ability to institute a more sensitive and selective program than the federal government, has been the basis for many arguments opposing the new proposal, although it is not possible to state confidently that health planning, PSROs, and state budget or rate review could form the basis for a national program.

In contrast to the local character of rate review, health planning, and the PSROs, the proposed Hospital Cost Containment Act, described in the next chapter, is essentially a federal program. The legislation only minimally involves state and local activities or concerns in its design. Moreover, it does not contain the data "feedback loops" implied by the regionally based programs, and, therefore, is more susceptible to concerns based upon the existing inadequate data base.

5 | A New Effort to Contain Hospital Costs

On April 25, 1977, early in his new administration, President Carter sent a message to Congress containing his proposals to improve the health care system. While noting that the United States spends more than any other country on health care ($160 billion in 1977), President Carter also pointed out that many individuals still lack adequate health care. Moreover, he stated that the cost of health care is rising so rapidly that it jeopardizes the nation's health goals and other important social objectives. The two administration proposals to deal with these problems were the Child Health Assessment Program, which was directed at assuring that low-income children receive regular, high quality primary and preventive care, and the Hospital Cost Containment Act of 1977.

> I am today proposing legislation which will limit the growth of the major component of health costs increases—rising hospital expenditures. The Hospital Cost Containment Act will restrain increases in the reimbursements which hospitals receive from all sources: Medicare, Medicaid, Blue Cross, commercial insurers, and individuals. The limit will be set by using a formula which not only reflects general inflation, but also extends to hospitals an additional allowance for improving their quality of care. Based on current trends, the limit for fiscal year 1978 will be approximately nine percent.
>
> The legislation will also impose a limit on new capital expenditures for acute care hospitals. The program will fix a national level for such expenditures below that of recent years and allocate new capital spending among the states by formula. With the assistance of local planning agencies, each state will determine which facilities merit new capital expenditures.[1]

The president then described the specific methods by which the bill would achieve the objectives of controlling hospital reimbursement and capital expenditures, and the newest effort to combat the entrenched ability of the medical care economy to generate increased costs had begun. The president opened for the offense by pointing out that:

> Without immediate action, the Federal government's bill for Medicare and Medicaid—which provide health care for our elderly and poor citizens—will jump nearly 23 percent next year, to $32 billion.
>
> Rising health care costs attack state and local governments as well. State and local Medicaid expenditures have grown from $3 billion in 1971 to $7 billion in 1976, forcing cutbacks which harm the low income recipients of the program.
>
> Unrestrained health costs also restrict our ability to plan necessary improvements in our health care system. *I am determined, for example, to phase in a workable program of national health insurance.* But with current inflation, the cost of any national health insurance program the Administration and the Congress will develop will double in just five years. [Emphasis added.]
>
> Finally, uncontrolled medical care spending undermines our efforts to establish a balanced health policy. Medical care is only one determinant of our people's health. The leading cause of death for Americans under 40 is motor vehicle accidents. The leading causes of death for older Americans—heart disease and cancer—are directly related to our working conditions and our eating, drinking, smoking, and exercise habits. We can better confront these broader health problems if we can limit the increases in soaring medical care costs.[2]

Perhaps in an effort to differentiate his new proposal from the Ford administration's proposal to limit Medicare reimbursement increases to 7 percent per year on a per diem basis, the president explained the rationale for covering all payers:

> To control escalating hospital costs, some have proposed to cap Medicare and Medicaid expenditures. Such a federal spending limit would encourage hospitals to reduce their services to low-income and elderly patients and to recoup rising expenses by increasing their charges to all other Americans. In contrast, the legislation I am proposing today reduces the growth in federal Medicare/Medicaid expenditures without imposing such severe new burdens on other purchasers of health services.[3]

That the program would impose no new burdens on other purchasers of health services appeared to be a confusing way of saying that the program will control all purchasers. Joseph A. Califano, Jr., secretary of Health, Education and Welfare, echoed the president's statements, but in a much less restrained fashion. "There is absolutely no competition among them....Hospitals have become over the years, many of them, quite obese....They are not trim."[4] In later comments, the secretary used phrases such as "gargantuan increases," "galloping cost increases." "intolerable escalation," and "inflation is on the rampage in the health industry" to describe the situation.[5] Continuing, Califano focused upon the impact of unrestrained hospital costs:

> Public opinion polls indicate that rising health care costs are among the top three domestic concerns of the American people—even ranking ahead of rising energy costs. This concern reflects a fundamental fact—rising health costs add significantly to burdens on the taxpayer, on the wage earner, and on those consumers who lack adequate health insurance protection.
>
> Each day American taxpayers pay $48 million for hospital care provided under Medicare and Medicaid.
>
> Private health insurance premiums have jumped 20–30 percent in the last year, cutting into most workers' take-home pay. Indeed Americans today must work more than one full month of every year to pay for their health care. It takes about two weeks wages to pay for hospital care alone. Higher health insurance premiums paid for fully or in part by employers drain off money that could be provided to workers in the form of higher wages and benefits.[6]

Confident of early passage, or at least making an effort to appear so, the administration transmitted the proposed legislation to Congress with an October 1, 1977 start-up date included in the bills. Further, the president had predicted the proposal's savings in his February 22 budget message to the Congress. According to HEW:

> The savings resulted from implementation of the Administration program would be enormous. In Fiscal Year 1978 alone, net savings would total $1.855 billion—including $578 million in Medicare funds, $143 million in Medicaid and $879 million in private funds.
>
> By 1980, net savings would nearly triple to $5.53 billion—including $1.755 billion under Medicare, $429 million under Medicaid, and $2.64 billion in private funds.[7]

After injecting a sense of urgency by enumerating the tremendous increases in hospital expenditures and by describing the predicted savings if the legislation were enacted in accordance with their timetable, administration officials attempted to explain why it would be reasonable and equitable to impose mandatory controls on the hospital care sector of the economy at a time when no controls were being imposed for other sectors. The former Economic Stabilization Program's Phases I and II may have been difficult, but they had general applicability to all sectors of the economy. The major controversy associated with ESP arose under Phases III and IV when controls had become selective, rather than universal. Moreover, President Carter's other major economic proposal, the Energy Program, proposed to *decrease* the degree of regulation on certain energy costs.

This is an especially important point in the context of HEW's statement that the Hospital Cost Containment Act was "a major component of the administration's overall anti-inflation program."[8] Yet on January 19, 1978, while the administration was still attempting to push the cost containment bill through the Congress, the president indicated in his State of the Union address that he was opposed to mandatory economic controls. "I do not believe in wage and price controls," he stated. "A sincere commitment to voluntary constraint provides a way— *perhaps the only way* [emphasis added]—to fight inflation without government interference." And he also asked that government, business, labor, and other groups "join in a voluntary program to moderate inflation by holding wage and price increases in each factor of the economy during 1978 below the average increase of the last two years."[9]

There are many structural differences in the hospital care industry which make it essentially immune to the inflation-restraining forces which hit other industries. Nevertheless, the administration was proposing something for hospitals which it clearly felt was inappropriate for other industries and, therefore, it was obligated to present a strong case as to why hospitals were different. The effort was begun by Secretary Califano:

> There is no incentive for hospitals to be efficient. The incentives that encourage the non-hospital sector of American industry to provide more and better goods and services to our American citizens are wholly absent in the hospital industry.
>
> —Hospitals operate on a cost-plus basis, the least efficient way to operate economically.
> —Hospitals operate on a sole source procurement basis, with doctors advising patients which hospital they must go to and the patient having limited freedom to choose among hospitals.
> —The user of the service rarely pays. Ninety percent of the hospital bills are paid by third party payers. Thus, the patient never has a sense of the exorbitant price of the service he receives.
> —The user of the service—the patient—does not choose the service. His doctor usually tells the patient what he needs. The current system of third party payers reimbursing hospitals for whatever the cost-plus, sole source price is has created a "spend-more, get-more" attitude. This attitude encourages hospitals to add expensive new facilities and technology, helter skelter, without regard to costs, and too often without evaluation of long-term quality implications.
> —The system operates to put every incentive for spending and few if any incentives for efficiency.[10]

Up to this point, the statements of the president and Secretary Califano were in general agreement with views held by many health care economists and policy analysts. The major points expressed about the inefficiency of hospitals, the improper incentives contained within the third party payment system, the utility of hospital care versus other health care efforts, and the rising opportunity costs of hospital care are in general accordance with the research reported in Chapter 3. Nevertheless, everyone appears to be in favor of cost control. The political problem arises because, "when we break it down to specific action, we get into fights."[11] The situation was no different with the Hospital Cost Containment Act of 1977.

The Introduction of Cost Containment Legislation

On April 25, 1977, the administration's Hospital Cost Containment bill was introduced in the House of Representatives as H.R. 6575 by Congressman Paul Rogers (D.-Fla.) and Dan Rostenkowski (D.-Ill.), and referred to the Subcommittees on Health of the Committees on Interstate and Foreign Commerce and on Ways and Means, chaired by Rogers and Rostenkowski, respectively. The following day the bill was introduced as S. 1391 in the Senate by Senators Edward Kennedy (D.-Mass.), William Hathaway (D.-Maine), and Wendell Anderson (D.-Minn.), and referred to the Subcommittees on Health of the Committees on Human Resources and on Finance, chaired by Senators Kennedy and Herman Talmadge (D.-Ga.), respectively.

Although the administration's proposal was the first cost containment legislation introduced in the 95th Congress, it was by no means to be the last. In evidence of the lack of consensus on how controls should be structured, five other major proposals were to be introduced in the next four months. Talmadge had been working on a proposal of his own and had in fact introduced a version of it (S. 3205) in the 94th Congress. His dedication to his own proposal, and his refusal to cosponsor or to facilitate the administration proposal's passage, had the potential of seriously hindering efforts to pass the administration bill. Taking an independent stance, Senator Talmadge introduced his much different proposal, S. 1470, on May 5, 1977.

The other four proposals were all based upon the administration bill, but made a series of changes which the sponsors felt were necessary to improve the original proposal. H.R. 8121, introduced by Rogers on June 30, 1977, added incentives for good performance by hospitals and proposed a new program to identify and close excess capacity. H.R. 8337, introduced by Rostenkowski on July 14, 1977, changed the formulation of the revenue cap and exempted all small hospitals. H.R. 8687, introduced by Congressman Tim Lee Carter (R.-Ky.) on August 2, 1977, and S. 1878, introduced July 18, 1977 by Senator Richard Schweiker (R.-Pa.) went much further in encouraging the formulation of state rate and budget review programs than had the administration's proposal. Nonetheless, it was the Carter administration's initiative which framed the debate and provided the focus on what types of controls were needed. A review of the basic provisions of the administration bill is a necessary prerequisite to understanding the congressional response to rising health care costs.

H.R. 6575 and S. 1391: Summary of Basic Provisions

The bill is divided into three parts. The first part directs the secretary of HEW to submit to Congress no later than March 1, 1978 (assuming an October 1, 1977 commencement of the program), a report recommending permanent reforms to increase efficiency, effectiveness, and quality of health care in the United States; these reforms would replace the transitional provisions of Title I of the act.

The second part, Title I, would establish a transitional hospital cost containment program to constrain the rate of increase in acute care hospital inpatient costs by limiting the average per admission reimbursement received by the hospital from Medicare, Medicaid, and Blue Cross; it would also limit average per admission charges received by the hospital from commercial insurers and self-payers, pending the permanent reforms developed by the secretary. Title II would establish a $2.5 billion limit on national hospital capital expenditures, and would require the secretary to establish a mandatory ceiling on the supply of hospital beds at four beds per thousand population and a standard occupancy rate of 80 percent. Areas of the country found to be out of compliance with the standards would generally not be allowed to build any hospital beds.

Title I: Start and Duration of Program

The program was to have started on October 1, 1977 and was to continue until Congress, acting upon the report of the secretary due March 1, 1978, designed and acted upon a permanent program.

Comment. A major problem was associated with the start-up date. Every hospital would have been under the revenue controls on October 1, regardless of where the hospital was in its accounting year. Only about 15 percent of all hospitals use an October 1 accounting year and, therefore, the majority of hospitals would have been subject to two different revenue limits in one accounting year. As for the "transitional" aspect of the program, the bill contained no definite termination date for the program, but only the vague assurances contained in the secretary's report on permanent reform.

Application of Revenue Limits

The proposed limitations on revenues would have applied only to *inpatient* revenues in approximately 6,000 short-term hospitals. Hospitals with an average length of stay of over 30 days were excluded. Also excluded were those hospitals receiving 75 percent or more of their non-Medicare revenue on a capitation basis from federally qualified health maintenance organization, hospitals less than two years old, and federal hospitals. The bill further proposed to exclude certain hospitals if the secretary found that exclusion was necessary to facilitate experimentation in other forms of cost containment under the Social Security Amendments of 1967 and 1972 or Section 1526 of the Public Health Service Act (Health Planning), or under certain state rate-setting programs.

Comment. The application of revenue limits appears to have demonstrated the administration's desire to use the cost containment bill to promote other federal health initiatives. The exclusion of outpatient costs was based upon the assumption that in so doing the bill would provide an incentive to shift services into the ambulatory setting, which is assumed to be a less expensive form of care. Similarly, the HMO exclusion seemed intended to provide hospitals with an incentive to participate in the federal HMO program. The legislation's facilitation of experiments and state programs is quite logical, considering the need to devise a permanent program; however, there was disagreement about how much latitude should be allowed the states in designing and operating their own cost containment programs. For example, organized labor tended to favor a federal program with uniform standards, while the Conference of State Legislatures tended to support the widest possible discretion for the states. More importantly, a great deal of concern was expressed by HEW about the ability of the states to perform adequately.

The exclusion of federal hospitals probably was more a political move than a policy decision, although the administration argued that federal hospitals were already under resource controls due to the congressional budgetary process which allocates funds to them. A more likely explanation is that opposition exists in Congress to any proposal that would place curbs on the use of resources by these hospitals; most federal hospitals are Veterans Administration facilities. Moreover, there were already four congressional committees involved in scrutinizing the bill, and the addition of controls on federal hospitals undoubtedly would have created further problems in obtaining approval of the bill. Neither the administration nor the congressmen wanted such a fight while also attempting to place controls on nonfederal hospitals.

Setting the Basic Revenue Limits

For each fiscal year beginning on October 1, 1977, the secretary of HEW would promulgate an inpatient hospital revenue increase limit equal to the rate of increase in the GNP deflator during the preceding 12-month period ending June 30, *plus* one-third of the *difference* between the actual annual increase in hospital expenditures *and* the annual increase in the GNP deflator during the two preceding calendar years. The GNP deflator is a measure devised by the Bureau of Economic Analysis of the Department of Commerce, and is derived by dividing current-dollar gross national product by constant-dollar gross national product; it is, therefore, a general measure of relatively pure inflation in the economy. The following illustration[12] provides an example of the process:

GNP deflator 7/1/76 to 6/30/77 minus
GNP deflator 7/1/75 to 6/30/76 $= 106 - 100 = 6\%$

Annual increase in hospital expenditure $= 1976$ over $1974 = 15\%$
Annual increase in GNP deflator: 1976 over $1974 = 6\%$
Basic limit: $6 + \frac{1}{3}(15 - 6) = 9\%$

The limit derived would be applied with adjustments for volume, to average per admission reimbursement from each third party cost payer, and to average charges per admission for the hospital accounting year ending in 1976 inflated by not more than 15 percent per year nor less than 6 percent per year to the effective date of the program. Essentially, each cost payer independently would calculate the average reimbursement per admission provided by that payer in the base year. Similarly, average per admission charges would be derived by dividing total charges, whether or not billed or paid, by total admissions attributable to charge payers. Each resultant figure would be adjusted for volume and inflated upward for each intervening year (or part thereof) between 1976 and the start-up year by adding the actual average increase in costs to each figure, although in no case could the adjustment be more than 15 percent or less than 6 percent. The prevailing inpatient hospital revenue increase limit would then be added to the figures derived for each class of payer to arrive at allowable reimbursement and allowable charges once the program began. The following illustration[13] provides an example:

Assume: Base Accounting Year end 6/30/76

Actual costs rose at an average monthly rate of 1% from 7/1/74 to 6/30/76.

No change in the rate of admissions existed during this time period and, therefore, the basic rate of 9% applies (¾% per month).

Calculation:

Allowance for inflation 6/30/76 to 10/1/77:
15 months × 1% = 15%

Limit applied from 10/1/77 to 6/30/78:
9 months × ¾% = 6.75%

	1976	Limit	Allowed
Medicare reimbursement per admission	$2,006	1.2175	$2,516
Medicaid reimbursement per admission	1,860	1.2175	2,265
Blue Cross reimbursement per admission	1,488	1.2175	1,812
Charges per admission	2,479	1.2175	3,018

Comment. An early issue arose about the design of the limit, and concerned the extent to which input prices in the hospital market basket would rise faster than the GNP deflator. Although the GNP deflator is thought to be the best economy-wide measure of pure inflation, the American Hospital Association has argued that prices for hospital inputs have been rising faster than prices in the general economy.[14] Although cost-push inflation independently does not have sufficient power to explain hospital inflation, controls based upon incorrect assumptions about input price inflation will be more stringent if the inflation measure is too low. This issue was not completely answered because of the lack of data; furthermore, it was overshadowed by more specific concerns about the design of the revenue limit.

Perhaps the most important concern was that the proposed revenue limit contained a "double ratchet" effect. This occurred because the limit actually declined over time for two reasons. First, the allowance for intensity increases (one-third of the difference between actual inflation and the GNP deflator) would decline because the program would cause actual hospital inflation to decline. Returning to the illustration above, in the first year of the program actual inflation was 15 percent and the GNP deflator equalled 6 percent. One-third of the difference equals 3, and the limit was 9. In the second year, actual inflation would have been reduced to about 11 percent due to the application of the limit plus additional adjustments for volume and exceptions. Therefore, one-third of the difference between actual hospital inflation and the GNP deflator, assuming it stayed constant, would be about 1.6 percent, and the resultant limit would be only about 7.6 percent. This process would continue and the limit would be brought closer and closer to the GNP deflator.

The second part of the effect occurs because the revenue limit would be applied annually in an additive manner to the 1976 base year revenues, rather than to the previous year's inpatient revenues. The effect would be that the actual year-to-year rate of increase would be substantially less than the administration was claiming it to be, as demonstrated in Table 5-1.

The double ratchet effect, therefore, meant that the proposed program was more stringent than had been stated. Recognizing that hospital revenues had been increasing at an *annual* rate of 15.6 percent, it was not at all clear that hospitals would be able to reverse the situation in such a short time period without serious disruptions in the production of their all-important services. Although the question of what level of support a society should allocate to the production of health care services is a social policy question and society is relatively free to decide what that level should be, it is not likely that the question can be settled by allowing increases which are less than the general level of inflation. It seems highly likely that the aggregate impact of these two effects would have done precisely that; the result would have been a net decrease in the percentage of GNP going to hospital care.

Moreover, even if one accepts completely the previous arguments about the existence of considerable excess services and capacity in the hospital industry, such excess is maldistributed, as are many health and medical care services in this country. The constraints proposed by the administration might have begun to shrink the excess due to the stringent nature of the proposed controls, but there was no guarantee that the controls would have had more impact on unneeded services than on needed ones. The administration proposed the same basic limit on every hospital without regard to established community need for such a facility, or to previous efforts by a hospital to save costs (thus lowering its base year revenue), or to the type of hospital. Clearly, those hospitals which had attempted to save money in the past by cutting out under-utilized or unneeded services would have found themselves hard pressed to comply with the program. Furthermore, some hospitals would need to continue providing the tertiary level or more esoteric services needed by only a few patients. It was not clear what tertiary level or regional referral medical centers would do in the face of the proposed controls, nor what would happen to a patient in need of a more expensive service if a hospital decided to omit it. Basically, the issue was summarized by Congressman Carter in a statement to the House of Representatives: "Hospitals and the problems they face are as varied as the diseases with which we become infected; and an effective cost containment system must have the ability, and the sensitivity, to deal with these variations."[15]

Table 5-1

Actual Year-to-Year Increase in Hospital Revenue Limits
Under H.R. 6575

	Assumed Price Deflator	*Hospital Revenue Increase Limit*	*Increase Over Base Year*	*Increase Over Previous Year*
FY 1978	6.1	8.7	8.7	8.7
FY 1979	6.2	9.3	18.0	8.6
FY 1980	5.4	7.6	25.6	6.4
FY 1981	5.0	7.1	32.7	5.7
FY 1982	5.1	7.0	39.7	5.3

Note: Base year assumed to be 1977

Source: Prepared by the Staff of the Subcommittee on Health and the Environment for use by the Subcommittee during consideration of H.R. 6575, September 1977, (processed).

Adjusting for Volume

Although the revenue limit was calculated on a per admission basis to avoid any incentive to increase length of stay inherent in a per day–based calculation, the administration further proposed to avoid incentives toward increased admissions and to provide incentives toward decreasing volume through the use of a patient-load adjustment. First, the basic limit would be adjusted for changes in the number of admissions only if admissions since the base year had increased by more than 2 percent or by less than 6 percent (or 10 percent in the case of smaller hospitals, i.e., those with fewer than 4,000 admissions per year). For increases above 2 percent and below 15 percent, or indefinitely for smaller hospitals, the total revenue limit would rise at a rate of 50 percent of the average allowable revenue per admission.

No increase in total revenue would be allowed for larger hospitals with volume increases over 15 percent, unless an exception was granted. Similarly, total revenue would be decreased by 50 percent of the average revenue per admission for decreases between 6 percent (10 percent for smaller hospitals) and 15 percent. Beyond 15 percent, revenues would be decreased by 100 percent of the average per admission revenue for each decrease in the number of admissions beyond 15 percent. Essentially, this approach provides that revenue per admission would increase if the number of admissions decreased, and it would decrease if admissions increased as shown in Table 5-2.

Comment. Although the patient-load adjustment appears complicated at first glance, it can be presented as a simple chart with the adjusted limit displayed for each volume level. Theoretically, it is based upon a recognition of the difference between average cost and marginal cost. The 50 percent reduction (or increase) in revenue per admission is based upon the assumption that variable costs equal 50 percent of average costs, and adding or subtracting that amount provides ample recognition of the hospital's fixed costs which do not vary with volume. Moreover, the use of the adjustment theoretically removes any incentives toward higher volumes since deletion of variable cost precludes the hospital from improving its operating margin as volume increases. Some concern was expressed by congressional committee members about the validity of the 50 percent measure as a proper reflection of variable costs, but HEW[16] claimed that its review of the literature revealed no measure of variable costs higher than 40 percent and, therefore, the proposed adjustment was actually on the generous side. Nevertheless, the "admission load formula" was to remain as a crucial point of contention during consideration of the bill.

Nonsupervisory Wage Increase Adjustment

The basic revenue increase limit could also be further adjusted, at the hospital's option, to "pass-through" wage increases granted to the hospital's nonsupervisory employees. The hospital would have had to provide the data necessary to verify the wage increases.

Percentage of total cost attributable to nonsupervisory wages = 40%
Percentage of total cost attributable to all other costs . . . . = 60%
Nonsupervisory wage increase . . . . = 10%
Basic limit . . . . =   9%

Substitute limit = $(.40 \times .10) + (.60 \times .09) = (.04) + (.054)$ = 9.4%

Table 5-2

Revenue Adjustments for Patient-Load Changes
Under H.R. 6575

	Admissions	Adjusted Limit	Revenue Per Admission	Total Revenue
Base Year	10,000	N/A	$1,000	$10,000,000
5% Admission Increase	10,500	5.3664%	1,054	11,067,000
1% Admission Increase	10,100	7.9212	1,079	10,900,000
Admissions Unchanged	10,000	9.0000	1,090	10,900,000
6% Admission Decline	9,400	15.9760	1,160	10,900,000
8% Admission Decline	9,200	17.2935	1,173	10,791,000

Note: "Adjusted Limit" is the allowable percentage increase in revenue per
admission with a 9 percent increase used as an illustration.

Source: Prepared by the Staff of the Subcommittee on Health and
the Environment for use by the Subcommittee during consideration of H.R. 6575, September 1977 (processed).

Comment. During subcommittee consideration of the bill, administration spokesmen stated that this provision was included because, under
the Economic Stabilization Program, hospitals had chosen to meet the
requirements of the controls by holding down the wages of lower level
employees. However, some evidence was presented that hospital workers' wages were actually higher than their counterparts in other industries, as noted in Chapter 3 in the discussion on labor. A more widely
accepted explanation for this proposal is that the labor unions, particularly the AFL-CIO, insisted upon it, although they were dissatisfied
with the optional character of the provision.[17]

Opponents of the pass-through component expressed concern that it
would interfere in the collective bargaining process since hospital
administrators would have little incentive to resist inappropriate wage
demands on the part of nonsupervisory workers. In addition, the
possibility exists that the pass-through would increase all wages through
a ripple effect as higher paid employees would press the hospital administration to keep salary differentials at the level existing before the
program went into effect.

There appears to be another problem in the structure of the pass-through. Since the provision was optional, it is possible that a hospital administrator could give nonsupervisory employees a large wage increase in one year, pass it through the revenue limits and then not use it the following year, allocating instead the entire revenue increase for that second year to nonwage components of the hospital budget. HEW later requested a "technical amendment" which remedied the problem, although technical amendments are not commonly meant to have as great an impact upon policy as did this one. Essentially, the amendment insured that if a hospital requested the wage pass-through for any year, wages would continue to be passed through for succeeding years.

Exceptions to the Revenue Limit

The proposed Hospital Cost Containment Act provided that a hospital could be granted an exception to the revenue limits by the secretary if the hospital had had an increase in admissions higher than 15 percent or if the hospital had instituted major changes in facilities or services, provided that the changes were found to be necessary and appropriate by the state health planning and development agency. In addition, it would be necessary for the hospital to demonstrate a poor financial position, defined as having a current ratio of assets to liabilities which the secretary estimated was less than that experienced by the lower 25 percent of hospitals covered by the program. In determining the general need for an exception, the secretary was required to take into account all sources of revenue, including philanthropy and locally raised tax dollars. If a hospital were to be granted an exception, it would be allowed only an increase in revenue such that its financial position would be maintained at a current ratio equal to that experienced by the lowest 25 percent of all hospitals. The hospital would also have to make itself available for an operational review by the secretary, and continuance of the exception was to be contingent upon the hospital's implementation of any recommendations made as a result of that review.

Comment. The exceptions process clearly was one place where the proposal contained provisions which were specific and sensitive to the circumstances of varied institutions. Considering the uniformity of the revenue limits and the wide variations among hospitals, it would seem logical to design an exception process that reduces the inequities associated with a uniform cap. The administration's bill did tie exceptions to the hospital's financial position and it also provided for a detailed scrutiny of the operation of hospitals granted an exception, although the review essentially meant that the secretary of HEW could dictate operational changes to the institution and this was an area of concern to many.

On a more negative side, the administration used an arbitrary measure for insolvency and further required that there be an increase in admissions beyond 15 percent or a change in facilities or services before an exception could be granted. On the one hand, therefore, a hospital experiencing financial difficulty, perhaps through no fault of its own, would not be eligible for an exception if it had not undergone the prescribed changes. On the other hand, an institution might find that no matter how justified an exception increase might be on the grounds of volume or service changes, it would not be reviewed unless it was threatened with insolvency. Clearly, the assumption was that it was preferable for hospitals to "spend down" their reserves before exception relief would be granted, although it was certainly possible that a hospital would choose instead to cut services—services which may have been essential to the well-being of the community served by the hospital. Although this possibility may have been remote, taking into account the normal incentives toward providing a full range of services and the existence of significant excess capacity, there was concern that the administration's bill provided no way to monitor or to avoid this problem.

The administration assumed, therefore, that the level of inefficiency is distributed fairly evenly among all hospitals, and that it would be large enough to insure that stringent resource constraints with little opportunity for exception relief would have little or no impact upon access to needed care or upon the range of quality of services provided.

Exemptions for State Programs

The bill provided exemptions for certain state programs as long as they met a series of fairly stringent requirements: (1) the state program must have been in operation for at least one year, and cover at least 90 percent of the hospitals included under the federal program; (2) the aggregate rate of increase for inpatient revenues must be contained at a rate not exceeding the rate promulgated under the federal program; (3) the program must have a plan acceptable to the secretary for recovering any excess revenue; and (4) the program must apply to all non-Medicare inpatient revenue. In a separate section, the proposed bill also exempted those state programs funded under federal rate-setting experiments authority contained in P.L. 90-248, P.L. 92-603, and P.L. 93-641.

Comment. It was apparent that the administration's bill did not envision any significant state effort, as evidenced by the requirement that state programs had to be in operation at least one year before becoming eligible for exemption from federal requirements. In including this requirement, the administration was essentially saying that it had little faith in the ability of the states to operate a tough program and, therefore, that the secretary of HEW would have to pass on the ability of each program after it had been in operation for at least one year. This is not a particularly unusual view on the part of the federal government, but it must be remembered that up to this point states had shown far more willingness to institute tough action on rising hospital costs than had the federal government.

The proposed bill further required that the rate of increase in state programs be no greater than the *promulgated* rate under the federal program. This was a significantly more difficult measure because the federal program actually allowed a higher rate, due to the effects of the wage pass-through, the volume adjustment, and the exceptions process. HEW originally estimated that if the revenue increase limit was 9 percent, actual allowable inflation would reach 10.8 percent.

Another interesting point was that of all of the states which were envisioned to be sufficiently experienced to meet the requirements (Connecticut, Maryland, Massachusetts, Washington, and perhaps New York), all but New York would qualify under the experimental provision. Many of New York's hospitals were participating in experiments and would have qualified for exemption; however, no experiment included the complete state.

Enforcement and Disclosure of Information

Enforcement of the provisions was fairly straightforward. The Medicare intermediary would be responsible for monitoring both cost reimbursement and charges. Reimbursement above the revenue increase limits would not be paid under Medicare and Medicaid. Overpayments by other third party cost reimbursers would be subject to a 150 percent tax on both the hospital and the payer. Since return of excess charges to patients charged individually was not practical, the tax would be levied on the hospital unless it placed the excess amount in escrow until the hospital experienced a shortfall in allowable charge revenue equal to the amount of the excess. Moreover, the secretary could also prevent a hospital or payer found to be in violation of the revenue increase limits from participating in Medicare, Medicaid, or the Maternal and Child Health programs.

The bill also provided that Health Systems Agencies investigate complaints made by a hospital that another hospital was "dumping" those patients for which it received a lower average reimbursement per admission, particularly Medicaid patients. If investigation proved that a hospital was guilty of "dumping," the secretary could exclude that hospital from federal reimbursement programs.

Hospitals would be required to submit certain information to the HSA including its semiprivate room rates, all cost reports submitted to third party cost payers, and its overall plan and budget as described under section 1861 (z) of the Social Security Act. The HSA would have been required to publish the information twice a year in a way which would allow comparisons among hospitals in the HSA's health service area. Again, noncompliance on the part of the hospital might lead to exclusion from the federal reimbursement programs at the discretion of the secretary.

Comment. Some congressmen were greatly concerned that the anti-dumping provision was too weak.[18] Obviously, there is a general incentive to increase revenue, and it would be expected that this would be true especially in the face of stringent revenue controls. Reducing the percentage of patients for whom reimbursement is low (Medicaid patients and certain self-payers prone to not paying their bills) and increasing the percentage of patients for whom reimbursement is high and reasonably assured (especially patients covered by private insurance) will increase total revenue. HEW countered by pointing out that this problem occurs regardless of the imposition of revenue controls, and that the structure of the system did not exacerbate the problem.[19] Nevertheless, the existence of the problem indicated that some investigational capability was necessary, although the HSA may not have been the proper unit.

Appeals Process

The bill provided an appeals process for those hospitals which were dissatisfied with determinations made by the secretary under the act. Appeals would go to an expanded Provider Reimbursement Review Board under procedures previously developed for the board's Medicare reviews.

Discontinuation of Services

As a means of insuring that hospitals did not attempt to improve their financial position by closing services or by allocating the costs of services to outpatient departments, the legislation provided that the revenue base would be reduced by the base year revenue attributed to services no longer being offered within (or allocated to) the hospital's inpatient services unless, in the case of discontinuance, the service was found to be unneeded by the regional health planning agency.

Comment. One problem immediately apparent in this provision is that it may remove the incentives to close out excess capacity, given that few of the regional health planning agencies are conducting appropriateness review at the present time. The provision would mean that the only services which the hospital would have an incentive to close would be those operating at a loss. In consideration of Roemer's law[20] (a larger supply generates higher utilization), and the existing ability of hospitals to raise revenue at will, it can be concluded that there *is* excess capacity which is not being operated at a loss. For this reason, it seems logical to provide the hospital with an incentive to close services, and thus reduce its cost, by allowing the hospital to retain some of the revenue lost due to closure.

Title II: Limitations on Hospital Capital Expenditures

The administration's proposal included a national limitation on capital expenditures, as well as limitations on revenue increases. The legislation proposed an aggregate $2.5 billion limit per year, apportioned initially among the states on the basis of population with subsequent adjustment for differences in construction costs, the need for facilities or modernization of existing facilities, and other appropriate factors.

Capital expenditure was defined as an expense not for operation or maintenance which changed bed capacity, substantially changed services, *or* exceeded $100,000. Capital expenditures were further limited by a national ceiling on the supply of beds of four beds per thousand population, and a national occupancy standard of no less than 80 percent. No hospital within a health service area which did not meet both these standards would be allowed to build any beds, except that one new bed could be built in areas in which two beds had been closed.

The provisions were to be enforced by state health planning and development agencies through the certificate of need process (see Chapter 4). No state would be allowed to issue a certificate of need to approve an expenditure in excess of the state's allocation under the $2.5 billion limit, or for an increase in beds, when the health service area was not in compliance with the supply and occupancy standards. The bill also would resolve existing differences in the certificate of need provisions contained in the Public Health Service Act and in Section 1122 of the Social Security Act.

Finally, the bill put more teeth into existing certificate of need laws by insuring that if a hospital in a state without an approved certificate of need program undertook a capital expenditure, the secretary was directed to reduce that hospital's federal reimbursement by an amount equal to ten times the amount of depreciation, interest, and return on equity capital attributable to that expenditure. Present law requires that the secretary exclude only the actual amount attributable to those capital costs in determining allowable reimbursement.

Comment. When considering the importance of capital expenditures in fueling the inflationary spiral in health care, restraints on those expenditures certainly make a great deal of sense. One problem with the administration's proposal was that the ceiling could not be defended because of its arbitrary nature, although it seemed to have been intended to halve present expenditure levels for other than beds, since HEW projects that $5 billion will be spent for purposes other than beds in fiscal 1978 (See Table 5-3). The ceiling did not seem to be based upon any objective assessment of need. The Department of Health, Education, and Welfare calculated that a $2.5 billion ceiling would reduce inflation in operating costs to the point necessary for hospitals to meet the 3 percent differential between allowable operating revenues under the program and the general rate of hospital inflation.[21] Unfortunately, because expenditures were already "in the pipeline," capital expenditures would exceed the $2.5 billion ceiling until 1981 and the revenue differential would be less than 3 percent by that date.

Another problem with the proposal was that the $2.5 billion ceiling only applied to reviewable expenditures, those meeting the thresholds specified in the certificate of need laws (generally expenditures over $100,000). It was not clear whether hospital capital expenditures would shift into nonreviewable areas. For example, a C.A.T. scanner recently came on the market for less than $100,000, leading to the suspicion that the manufacturer was attempting to avoid the certificate of need laws and the proposed ceiling.

Finally, the allocation process failed to take into account any differences in need among the states. If it is assumed that the distribution of facilities and services is closely approximated by the distribution of beds, the existence of the national range among states extending from 2.2 beds per thousand population to 6.7 beds per thousand leads to the conclusion that a distribution of capital expenditures based upon population alone is insufficient. Although the administration's proposal required that a more sophisticated allocation system be used in the second fiscal year of the program, HEW's previous tardiness in meeting other similar requirements would cause one to view the implied promise of a better allocation system with some skepticism.

Table 5–3

Comparsion of Hospital Capital Expenditures in
Fiscal Year 1978 Under Current Policy and Under the
$2.5 Billion Ceiling

(In $ billions)	FY 1978—Under Current Policy	FY 1978—Under Administration's Proposal		
	New CON's[4] & Work on Previously Approved Projects	New Spending (includes Expenditures Under New CON's)	Work on Projects Approved Before Imposition of Ceiling	Combined Total Spending
New beds[1]	1.8	—	1.8	1.8
Other construction and modernization[2]	4.0	1.0[5]	2.0	3.0
Equipment over $100,000 per project[3]	1.0	.5	—	.5
Total requiring CON approval	6.8	1.5	3.8	5.3
Total not requiring CON approval	1.2	1.2	—	1.2
Total Capital Expenditures	8.0	2.7	3.8	6.5

[1]Spending attributable to new beds is assumed to have been approved and initiated three years previously; the total expenditure is recorded for the year the project is completed.

[2]Spending for construction and modernization not attributable to new beds is assumed to take place as follows: one-half of the projects are assumed to have been approved one year previously, with all of the expenditures for a particular project recorded the year the project is completed. The other half of the projects are assumed to have been approved in the same year that they are completed and recorded.

[3]Spending for equipment and technology is assumed to have been approved in the same year it is completed and recorded.

[4]CON's = Certificate of Need

[5]In keeping with footnote 2 above, another $1.0 billion will be approved, but will be actually spent in the next fiscal year. This brings the total for newly approved CON's in FY 1978 up to the $2.5 billion allowed under Title II of the proposal.

Source: Office of Research and Statistics, Social Security Administration and Congressional Budget Office. Provided to the Subcommittee on Health and the Environment for use during consideration of H.R. 6575, 1977 (processed).

Conclusions

In a general sense the administration's proposal was in line with the theoretical conclusions reached in Chapter 3. The proposal rejected the cost-push theories by basing the revenue increase upon the GNP deflator, and by making the wage pass-through optional. It clearly assumed that the extent of unneeded services and excess utilization was great enough to withstand reductions in the rate of increase in hospital revenue and in capital expenditures. Moreover, the proposal recognized the important role of the provider by assuming that the imposition of the revenue cap would force hospital administrators and medical staffs into making the hard choices necessary to increase efficiency in the production of health care services. This point was further recognized by assuming that through restraints on revenue, provider incentives toward a higher quantity of care and a higher style of care would be lessened, thereby slowing consumer demand.

Perhaps the most important point is that the administration's bill recognized that the inflationary spiral in hospital costs is unjustified in the face of a great deal of evidence suggesting that hospital care is not providing the benefits expected as a result of the increased investment in it. Unfortunately, the legislation proposed to apply these concepts in a vague and nonspecific fashion to a highly important social commodity.

Although it is clear that constraints on resources (as in HMOs) can cause providers to make different decisions about the quantity or intensity of the care they provide, it is not clear that those restraints can be applied in an arbitrary manner. Similarly, although it can be stated that there is significant excess bed capacity existing within the system, and little need in most areas for new construction, there may be areas where capacity is too low. The combined effect of the administration's proposed capital expenditures limitation and the tight exceptions process for the proposed revenue limitation might mean that those areas truly in need would not be able to obtain any new facilities.

Overlying all of the difficulties with the nonspecific approach of the bill is that the theoretical base for the bill is not widely known nor generally accepted by observers of the health care system. As the next chapter describes, it is not all that difficult to attack the administrations's proposal if the audience is unaware of the studies and data which bear out the conclusions reached earlier about inefficiency, duplication, overutilization, and unnecessary increases in costs. Moreover, opposition becomes much easier when the proponents of the proposed constraints do not provide needed data, or do not have the specific data necessary to state with certainty that the program will not have negative impact on the production of health care services.

Finally, even if a politician swallows his or her concerns and accepts the argument that in any case the program is temporary and will be replaced by a sophisticated methodology which will deal with those specific and, in light of the paucity of definitive data, justifiable concerns about impact, it would be helpful to have some idea of the shape of that permanent program and the time it will take to produce it. The administration's proposal provided no such information, and when it is considered that HEW delivered the National Health Planning Guidelines 15 months after the law *required* the department to deliver them, there was almost no assurance that the permanent program would be designed within a reasonable length of time.

6 | Reactions to the Proposal

Special Interest or Public Interest?

The reaction to the introduction of H.R. 6575, the Hospital Cost Containment Act of 1977, was immediate and generally negative. Alexander McMahon, president of the American Hospital Association, termed the bill "inequitable in design, wrong in concept, and impossible to administer," and further stated, "Its enactment would seriously jeopardize the present and future ability of hospitals to provide quality care to the American people."[1] Michael Bromberg, director of the Federation of American Hospitals (the for-profit hospitals), went even further: "If Congress votes to place a ceiling on hospital revenues and on hospital-based technology, then Congress will be voting to establish itself as the moral judge of the dollar value of increased life spans, fewer fatal heart attacks, reduced infant mortality, significant survival rates for cancer patients, and every life saving device or technique."[2]

In this way the two largest and most important hospital lobbyists forced Congress into the central dilemma associated with efforts to impose restraint on hospital cost increases. On the one hand, Congress was being asked to consider a specific, detailed piece of legislation designed to control hospital revenue. On the other hand, those controls were intended to apply to an industry whose product is widely accepted as vitally needed; but the level of resources necessary to achieve society's goals for that industry, improved health status, is ill-defined and poorly understood.

Congressmen appear to be much like any other nonprofessional consumers in their understanding of health care services, and in their views toward the production of those services. Much as most consumers rely upon their doctors or other health care professionals to define for them which services they need, Congress frequently relies upon the Washington representatives of the health care industry for information on the state of that industry. This is not to say that individual congressmen, particularly on the health subcommittees, are unsophisticated about the dynamics of the industry—especially inflationary cost increases. Problems do arise, however, when the health care industry claims that proposed restraints on its resources will be detrimental to needed health care services or quality of care, two very ill-defined terms. When industry lobbyists make these claims, essentially taking for themselves the role of guardians of the public's interest in quality health care, there is very little in the way of a countervailing force which states that the public's interest is not served by continuous increases in intensity of short-term acute care or by capital expansion which lowers overall occupancy rates or results in duplication of expensive services.

Unfortunately, members of the public, as individuals, are protected from the consequences of inflation in hospital costs through the third party payment system. Moreover, each *individual* citizen has an incentive to support the *individual* institution from which he or she conceivably may purchase health care services at some point in the future, and almost no incentive to curtail the amount of resources going to that institution. Even though the public might support cost containment in a general sense, when it comes down to a specific proposal which attempts to constrain the increase in resources going to a specific institution, public support for the proposal tends to evaporate.

An interesting way to view this situation is to think in terms of the overall goal of the health care system, better health. Society, or its legislative representatives, may be unhappy and uncomfortable as health care expenses come due and payable. Nevertheless, it is hard not to pay for them when the people on whom society has always depended for information about health care claim that payment of the bill is the only way the goal of better health can be achieved. The result of this situation is that representatives of the health care industry can claim that it is they who are protecting the public interest, while Congress is only selfishly protecting the federal budget. Although it is clear that industry lobbyists represent a special interest, the ill-defined nature of the system and the lack of definite support for cost containment from the public have caused Congress to proceed cautiously in passing legislation which these interests oppose.

The Opposition: Players and Their Response

The first step in the legislative process is subcommittee hearings, and three of the four subcommittees to which H.R. 6575 and S. 1391 were referred moved quickly in scheduling hearings. In the House of Representatives, the Commerce Health Subcommittee (chaired by Rogers) and the Ways and Means Health Subcommittee (chaired by Rostenkowski) held joint hearings beginning May 11, 1977. The Senate's Human Resources Health Subcommittee (chaired by Kennedy) commenced its hearing on May 24, 1977, while the Finance Health Subcommittee (chaired by Talmadge) did nothing at this point.

Although these hearings constituted an important part of the legislative deliberations on cost containment, they are the least important component of the whole process. This relative lack of importance results from the fact that, in this case, over 50 individual witnesses appeared during the two sets of hearings, each with a statement. The statements often overlapped, and each day of hearings was quite long and often tedious in the extreme. It is difficult for congressional staff who specialize in health care matters to remember and keep separate each individual statement, much less congressmen who are concerned with many legislative matters other than health care issues. For this reason, lobbyists who are interested in getting their message across know that they must return again and again to discuss the points originally presented at the hearings with staff and with the congressmen. Although the hearings give each individual or group a chance to present a public position on the matter at hand, it is the discussion of those views in the privacy of a congressional office which has greater impact upon proposed legislation. The custom of visiting congressional offices confers a large advantage on those organizations which maintain well-financed, well-staffed lobbyists in Washington who have the time to sit and talk with staff and with members of Congress, to provide technical assistance, and generally to promote a collegial relationship between themselves and congressional decision makers. In the case of hospital cost containment, most of this activity was conducted by representatives of the health care industry, thereby making their position on the proposed legislation the one most clearly transmitted to Congress. The next section describes the positions, and more importantly, the actions taken by each of the major groups in their attempts to defeat or substantially modify the president's proposal.

American Hospital Association (AHA)

Virtually all of the 6,500 private hospitals in the United States belong to the AHA and, therefore, the association justifiably claims to speak for all private hospitals. In actual practice the membership is diverse and many member hospitals also belong to other lobbying organizations which some hospitals feel better represent their specific interest.

Examples of these special interest groups are the Federation of American Hospitals (FAH), the National Council of Community Hospitals (NCCH), and organizations representing Catholic, Protestant, osteopathic, teaching, and other hospitals with a specialized focus. Nonetheless, AHA was able to mount an effective effort against the proposed cost containment legislation.

The association's general tack was to claim that most cost increases in hospital care were justified and outside the control of the hospital; its major point was that hospital inflation is a form of cost-push inflation because the items in the hospital market basket were inflating at a faster rate than items in the general economy. Although the administration countered with evidence developed by the Council on Wage and Price Stability, which indicated that only about one-half of cost increases are attributable to price factors,[3] AHA could point to an "800 percent" increase in malpractice premiums in the last seven years. This is a phenomenon of which many congressmen are aware, although AHA did not mention that regardless of tremendous increases, malpractice premiums usually amount to slightly less than 1 percent of the total budget of a hospital.

AHA also pointed out that increased demand for services, modernization and maintenance of service capacity, as well as new government regulations concerning reporting requirements, safety code compliance, and minimum wages all serve to increase operating costs. This last point was especially effective as AHA pointed out that in New York State the Hospital Association found in its 1976 *Report of the Task Force on Regulation* that "40 federal agencies, 96 state agencies, 18 city and county agencies, and 10 voluntary and quasi-public groups—a total of 164 agencies—regulate 109 areas of hospital operation. Of the 109 areas, 82 are monitored by at least 10 different agencies."[4]

In general, AHA avoided overt efforts to take advantage of congressional unease about the effects of resource constraints on needed hospital care; however, it did point out that "intensification of services" resulting from "our ability to treat patients today for which previously there existed no capability for definitive care"[5] had a large effect on hospital costs. HEW countered by stating that many of the increases were "excessive and unnecessary,"[6] but the problem facing Congress was that presently there is no good way to measure which increases are necessary and which are not. The contradictions inherent in AHA's position were not lost on every member, as attested to by the following exchange between Leo Gehrig, M.D., an AHA senior vice president, and Senator Kennedy:

Dr. Gehrig: There has been a development of increasing sophistication of technology and the ability to do more in a limited time. A day in a hospital is unlike a day in the hospital 10 years ago.

Sen. Kennedy: That may very well be true, but we don't know what the health implications of that are.

Gehrig: I think, Senator, one can debate that, but I think one only need look at some of the activities, to view the fact that we are now doing things in both the prolongation of life, the relief of pain and suffering that we couldn't do 10 years ago.

And I think it is well enough to challenge it in broad perspective. But I think it is also very defensible to say that hospitals, by these actions, are improving the quality of life.

Sen. Kennedy: Why aren't you doing that? Why don't you do an assessment in terms of the health implications, and why aren't we able to examine from a public policy point of view in terms of these issues, in terms of what this new technology really means....

To tell us that a day in the life of a hospital is a lot different today doesn't really help us very much—in terms of our responsibilities, of saying that we have decided that in this area of technology, this is what this particular equipment is going to mean in terms of improving quality of health, this is what it is going to mean in terms of infant mortality, expenditures in this are going to improve the quality of the American people.[7]

Dr. Gehrig went on to state that increases in health manpower had also added significantly to the total health bill. Senator Kennedy countered by asking:

Where does that show? How can you show that increased numbers of personnel have really improved the quality of care? No question that you have increased dramatically the numbers of personnel in terms of the various hospitals—but how can you show us what that has meant in terms of improving health, and at what cost?[8]

Although AHA was unsuccessful in persuading Senator Kennedy that intensity increases were always needed and proper, most congressmen do not share Senator Kennedy's interest in the health care field. A more representative statement would be that of Congressman B.F. Sisk of California:

Advances in medical technology have made possible new methods of treatment which can save lives, and when an individual is struck by illness or accident, he or she expects the best care possible. Our new methods of diagnosis and treatment, however, are costly, and a real factor in the rapid increase in the cost of medical care are the additional and expensive tests and procedures done by costly skilled technicians with advanced equipment.[9]

AHA claimed that its position was a more responsible approach in terms of controlling hospital costs than that of the administration. Partially responsible for the success of this claim was that AHA consistently pointed out that it supported health planning and certificate of need, and moreover, that it supported state rate review programs. In order to advance this claim, AHA concentrated much of its lobbying effort on pointing out the technical inconsistencies and inequities associated with the administration's proposal. This effort was greatly assisted by the AHA's hiring of a former Medicare official, Irwin Wolkstein, who is very familiar with the intricacies of health care financing and hospital accounting, and who enjoys wide respect on Capital Hill. As noted by Dr. Stuart Shapiro, a member of the staff of the Kennedy subcommittee, "on the technical level, Wolkstein has been most helpful. The AHA opposes the bill, but it has been willing to say, 'we are opposed, but if you plan to act anyway, we will suggest changes that will make the measure easier to administer.' "[10]

In meetings with congressmen and congressional staff, persons such as Gehrig, Wolkstein, and AHA's President Alexander McMahon and its Legislative Division Chief Michael Hash, voiced their concern about technical problems with the proposed legislation, and, in a very responsible fashion, offered their suggestions as to how the legislation could be improved.

Among the issues raised by AHA was that the controls proposed by H.R. 6575/S. 1391 were in fact retroactive. This was because the revenue limit would have been applied retroactively in hospitals with fiscal years ending at times other than September 30. For example, a hospital with a calendar year fiscal period would be subject to a maximum annualized inflation rate of 15 percent between January 1, 1977 and October 1, 1977 (the program's planned start-up date), and a maximum rate of 9 percent for the last quarter of the year. The problem was that when the hospital planned its 1977 budget, it had no way of knowing that the revenue limit was going to be imposed. Therefore, to the extent that a hospital's planned budget was above the allowable rate, it might have to make drastic cuts in its revenue budget in that last quarter to meet the mandatory revenue limitations.

AHA was also the first to point out the effects of the double ratchet (discussed in the preceding chapter), as well as the effect of the administration's proposal that state rate review programs meet a stiffer test than the federal program. AHA also hit hard on the question of why a program being billed as "transitional" contained no time limit, a point of significant concern when it is considered that new legislation would be required to terminate the proposed revenue limitations and capital expenditure limitations. Given the problems in getting the hospital cost containment bill passed, and the amount of time consumed, AHA was certainly justified in its skepticism about the length of the program.

Besides the effective work of the association's Washington staff in proposing changes to the administration proposal, AHA also enlisted the support of the many potentially influential hospital trustees and administrators around the country to exert pressure on Congress in defense of AHA's point of view. AHA periodically publishes a "President's Letter" and "Washington Alerts" to advise members on the status of health care legislation; it also conducts a weekly nationwide conference call between the Washington office and the 50 state hospital association chief executives. In an August 1977 "President's Letter," AHA President McMahon urged members to speak with their representatives in Congress during the August recess and asked that they

> point out the basic problem with the Carter proposal and the oppressive aspects of its various provisions. The basic problem is that a limitation on inpatient revenues related to the cost of living will reduce hospitals' ability to expand services to meet the medical needs of patients and will in some institutions reduce those services.
>
> Finally, you must seize every opportunity to explain why hospital costs are rising—the inflation in the rest of the economy; the susceptibility of hospitals to those parts of the economy that are themselves rising faster than the cost of living, like energy, malpractice insurance, and food: and the need to apply advances in medical science to the care of your patients.[11]

Needless to say, a large number of letters making precisely the points included in McMahon's statement began arriving in congressional offices, and a significant increase in requests from hospital representatives for appointments with congressmen was noted by congressional staff.

Although AHA changed its tactics at a later point in the process, these early efforts were quite successful; this is shown by the response to AHA's points embodied in a later version of H.R. 6575 and S. 1391 described in the following chapter.

Other health industry lobbyists did not choose to take the same course as did AHA; instead, they chose mainly to accuse the Congress and the administration of a lack of concern for health care and health status for even proposing that increases in costs be restrained. Nonetheless, in consideration of the lack of progress in passing this legislation, it cannot be said that they were less successful than AHA in efforts to block the bill. The most important of these groups was the for-profit hospitals.

The Federation of American Hospitals (FAH)

The for-profit hospitals lobby, The Federation of American Hospitals (FAH), has been termed the most aggressive health lobby in Washington,[12] and its executive director Michael Bromberg was described by an unnamed congressional health staffer as "the single most effective health lobbyist operating today."[13] The federation's arguments against the administration's proposal generally followed the same lines as AHA's arguments, but tended to employ stronger language. For example, "if the HEW plan were not so serious and so potentially dangerous to our nation's health, we would have to say it was absurd."[14] FAH also maintained that the hospital has little control over the number of services provided within a hospital: "This legislation would impose a ceiling on reimbursement to the hospital for costs incurred as the result of physician-ordered services. This leads hospitals into a Catch 22 position in which one law would require an institution to deliver a medical service while another law would penalize the institution if it delivered the service."[15] Again, Senator Kennedy was ready with an answer to the industry's argument, noting that "hospital administrators have extremely broad authority... affecting a whole range of different services."[16] But the FAH argument makes a great deal of intuitive sense to those who are unfamiliar with the evidence cited above and experience under Phases II and III of the Economic Stabilization Program which shows that hospital administrators do have an impact upon the volume of services provided in their institutions even though physicians are directly responsible for ordering services.

Other Hospital Lobbyists

Several other organizations besides AHA and FAH presented testimony at the hearings on cost containment, although none mounted as extensive a lobbying effort as did these two organizations. Other groups included the American Protestant Hospital Association, the American Catholic Hospital Association, the Council on Teaching Hospitals, the National Council of Private Psychiatric Hospitals, the National Council of Community Hospitals, as well as representatives of individual hospitals. Like that of FAH, their basic appeal was that the proposed cost containment bill would unnecessarily and inappropriately curtail the quality of care. A representative statement is that of the American Catholic Hospital Association: "We predict that in general H.R. 6575 will dramatically reduce the quality and scope of services rendered.... We have concluded that H.R. 6575 would specifically penalize the sick, the poor, the terminally ill, the aged—those whom our members have particularly pledged themselves to serve."[17]

Other hospital representatives testified about their special concerns with the proposed legislation with, for example, representatives of teaching hospitals pointing out that they were different from the nation's other hospitals and, therefore, should not be subject to the same constraints.[18] Another point made by representatives of HMO hospitals such as Kaiser, was that they were already cost effective and, therefore, should not be included in the program.[19]

An interesting statement was offered by the National Council of Community Hospitals (NCCH), an organization with only 65 member hospitals. NCCH President John Horty stated during hearings that "NCCH recognizes and endorses the need for immediate cost control measures. At the same time we believe structural reform is so important it should not be subordinated to a cost control program that could well become a permanent control system."[20] In addition, Horty explained that "it [H.R. 6575] could just as easily be labeled the Quality Containment Act of 1977 or the Innovation Containment Act of 1977 as the Cost Containment Act of 1977. As a *proposal* it does serve to open the dialogue. As *law,* however, it could close the debate for the foreseeable future."[21]

NCCH urged that, instead of the administration's proposal, a freeze be instituted for 24 months on increases in hospital employment and on hospital capital expenditures. Also, the NCCH proposed that compensation for the physician, as well as for the hospital, be reduced if a PSRO found an admission or continued stay unnecessary. During the 24-month period, NCCH proposed that a national debate be conducted on the components of a permanent control system.

NCCH's proposal was introduced by request on July 13, 1977 by Congressman John Duncan of Tennessee as H.R. 8295, and the NCCH provided the Congress with a detailed justification written by health economist Paul Feldstein of the University of Michigan.[22] Although NCCH claimed that the dollar savings would be equal to those expected under the administration's proposal, the claim was based upon the assumption that in the absence of NCCH's proposal, increases in full-time equivalent personnel and in capital expenditures would continue at the present rate. The justification also assumed that nonlabor- and noncapital-associated expenditures would not expand at any faster rate when NCCH's proposed controls were imposed. NCCH is a relatively small organization and appears not to command the attention from

HEW or the Congress that AHA or FAH can claim. Thus, NCCH's proposal never received the scrutiny that it perhaps deserved, and the information necessary to answer these questions was never forthcoming. Nevertheless, it was intriguing to see a hospital group proposing "its own system of controls as a means of reducing controls."[23]

American Medical Association (AMA)

No comment on health care lobbying would be complete without mentioning the American Medical Association (AMA), the largest single special interest contributor of campaign funds to House and Senate candidates. In its testimony before the congressional committees, the AMA was in general philosophical agreement with AHA noting, for example, the effects of inflation outside of the hospital industry and the lack of a termination date for a "transitional" program.[24] The AMA hit hardest on the Title II capital expenditure limitations, stating that the limitations were a "clear example of federal control over the community."[25] This was not an unexpected position because the AMA consistently has opposed the health planning act, partially because of the implied federal controls contained within it. In general, the AMA's statement was restrained and avoided for the most part the more strident claims about the negative impact of cost containment on health status. Moreover, AMA lobbyists were relatively quiescent during the early deliberations, and did not become active until it was proposed in a later bill to extend the certificate of need program to physicians' offices, a proposal with a more direct impact upon AMA's constituency.

The Opposition: Conclusions

AHA, FAH, and later in the process, AMA, were the major voices speaking in opposition to the administration's proposal. Other groups were involved in the process but generally concerned themselves with responding to only one or two specific issues. Besides those mentioned above, other important concerns represented included: the medical equipment manufacturers, who were frankly concerned about the effects of the bill on their markets;[26] the National Association of Health Services Executives, who were concerned about the effects of the bill on public general hospitals;[27] and various individual provider representatives including, for example, a radiologist concerned about the effects of the capital expenditure limitation on the distribution of C.A.T. scanners.[28]

Opposition lobbyists perform an important service by providing information to staff and to congressional members; in turn, congressmen and their staff must insure to the best of their ability that the information is correct and, if necessary, that opposite views are presented. Part of the problem with passing the hospital cost containment bill has been that many of the specific criticisms of the bill made by health care lobbyists were justified and could not be ignored. As the next chapter relates, many of the points raised by lobbyists were answered in subsequent drafts of the proposed legislation. Nonetheless, problems identified with the original proposal provided the opposition with a platform from which to attack the bill and, therefore, caused the bill to be seen as poorly conceived legislation due to the original, justifiable criticism directed toward it.

Aside from the general point that any resource constraints would interfere with the production of needed, high quality health care services, the following is a summary of the opposition's concerns about the administration's proposal:

1. The lack of a time limit in a program termed "transitional."
2. The retroactive nature of the revenue limits.
3. The double ratchet effect of the revenue limit.
4. The nonspecific nature of the revenue limits. Specifically, opposition lobbyists pointed out that there is a great deal of variation among hospitals and that application of the same percentage limit was inherently unfair, given that variation. Moreover, lobbyists noted that the percentage limitation penalized hospitals which had been cost-conscious in the past since 9 percent of a "fat" budget involved more dollars than did 9 percent of a "lean" budget.
5. The application of the cap by class of purchaser. Opposition lobbyists noted that not all payers paid the same rate. Therefore, losses incurred due to one payer such as Medicaid refusing to allow a 9 percent increase, or losses caused by increases in the percentage of admissions covered by the lower paying payer, could not be compensated for by increasing charges to other payers, as would be the common practice now.
6. The exceptions process. Lobbyists claimed that it was too "tight" and that hospitals would be threatened with insolvency before they would become eligible for an exception.
7. The limited nature of the state exemption and the fact that state programs would have to meet a more stringent test than did the federal program.
8. The capital expenditure limitation. Lobbyists argued that the $2.5 billion cap would not be justified in any way and that it had no relationship to the need for capital expansion. Moreover, most lobbyists stated that the health planning process was a sufficient control on unneeded capital expenditures.

These concerns were raised by the opposition lobbyists again and again in private meetings, at conferences in the hall during committee meetings, in letters from constitutents, and in other ways. Arrayed against this significant effort were the White House and HEW, and whatever research congressional staff were able to develop. Missing was any significant lobbying on the part of groups which could reasonably have expected to benefit from cost containment efforts, i.e., the public, Blue Cross, the private insurance companies, large employers, labor, and state and local governments. Instead, these groups seemed content with making statements at the hearings and lobbying for some specific concern. The job of actually getting Congress on record in favor of some form of restraint in health care cost increases, therefore, generally was left to HEW and the president.

Supporters

During the congressional hearings on hospital cost containment many witnesses stated their general support for the administration's proposal, although some agreed with Bernard Tresnowski of Blue Cross that, "a transitional revenue limitation program appears to be a viable, though far from ideal, course of action."[29] The National Association of Counties (NACo) echoed Blue Cross's general support for the bill but noted its concerns that the anti-dumping provisions of the bill were not strong enough. Given that counties are the major sponsors of hospitals in which most low-income Medicaid and non-sponsored patients are treated, NACo wanted H.R. 6575/S. 1391 to "guarantee that no hospital reduce its share of care to 'unprofitable' patients."[30]

Perhaps the most interesting position of the groups who favored the bill but had specific concerns about it, was that of the labor unions. For example, Marc Stepp of the United Auto Workers stated, "H.R. 6575 is an important step in overcoming the inertia which has prevented needed change in America's health system. Runaway health costs have been taking billions of dollars needlessly from the pockets of American health care consumers. By proposing new controls on hospital revenues, capital outlays, and further encouragement of health maintenance organizations, an appropriate beginning is made."[31] Bert Seidman of the AFL-CIO asserted that one of the strengths of the proposed legislation was in providing "a ceiling on total hospital revenues. This comprehensive approach would contain not only hospital charges but also excessive utilization of hospital beds and extravagant use of personnel and capital resources, some of which is of marginal value in diagnosing and curing disease."[32]

Joined by the American Federation of State, County, and Municipal Employees, the United Mine Workers, the Service Employees International Union, and the National Union of Hospital and Health-Care Employees, the unions parted company with the administration on the question of the wage pass-through. Their basic objection was that the administration had made the pass-through optional for the hospital, and labor felt it should be mandatory. In support of their position they quoted from the 1977 staff report of the Council on Wage and Price Stability on the rapid rise in hospital costs written by Martin Feldstein: "had earnings of hospital workers risen no faster than the average for all private, uniform production workers, the annual rate of increase in daily hospital costs would have been only about one percentage point lower."[33] Stated another way, "total labor costs were the source of only about one-tenth of the annual increase in average costs per patient day."[34] For this reason labor contended that nonsupervisory wages should be "totally taken out of the picture."

On the other hand, the Health Insurance Association of America (HIAA) also testified in favor of the bill, but against the wage pass-through. It is interesting that HIAA was using the same Council of Wage and Price Stability report in defense of its point of view! HIAA had provided the comparative tables from the Council's report for the record and pointed out that:

> Hospital worker wages are not only roughly comparable, but they are increasing at a more rapid rate, 7.9% since 1970 as compared with 6.5% for private non-farm workers. This is of particular concern since the number of FTE employees per patient day has been climbing steadily. Hence, the combined effect of rapidly increasing wage rates and incentives to substitute labor (without the cap) for other factors (subject to the cap) undercuts the intended effect of the cost containment program.
>
> The wage pass-through provision could be expected to take considerable pressure off hospital administrators in negotiating wage agreements with nonsupervisory workers. While pressure on the management side is declining, workers can be expected to press for the maximum possible increases before the Secretary of HEW reevaluates the pass-through provision in 18 months [as required by the bill]. The almost certain result will be higher wage rates for nonsupervisory workers than would have been the case without the pass-through.[35]

The technical basis, as opposed to the philosophical and emotional basis, for the different views on the relative status of hospital workers was that the AFL-CIO presented data developed by the Bureau of Labor Statistics which show differentials between hospital and other workers, while HIAA was presenting Council on Wage and Price Stability data. The two are based upon different occupational definitions. Nevertheless, the council's definitions are more recent, and the findings are in line with other research by Martin Feldstein[36] and data developed by the Maryland rate review commission.[37] Moreover, it is unusual to use the conclusions of a study while denying the veracity of the data upon which those conclusions are based, as the unions appear to have done in this case.

The labor unions and the private health insurers found themselves on different sides of another major issue raised by supporters of the cost containment bill, that is, the question of how much latitude states should be allowed in running their own cost containment programs. Labor favored a stringent approach, while the health insurers proposed that the federal government should not only allow states to develop their own programs, but that federal support should be provided to encourage such development. HIAA took this position because of its concern about the nonspecific nature of the administration's proposal[38] and because of its belief that "state prospective budget review and rate approval systems can accomplish this goal. In Connecticut and Maryland it has proved that costs can be controlled without adversely affecting the quality of care. It offers the local expertise and knowledge that a Federal system could never achieve. It makes possible a more sophisticated, in-depth review of a particular hospital operation than could a Federal system. And as a permanent solution it offers the flexibility needed to become an extremely effective regulatory process."[39] HIAA, joined by the National Conference of State Legislatures and other witnesses, emphasized the point that controls on reimbursement should be tied with health planning programs and utilization review and quality assurance programs. Spokespersons stated "that the present planning law and the professional standards reviewed organizations' efforts will be severely limited in their impact unless they are coordinated with prospective budget analysis. The bill must clearly spell out the need for interaction between these processes." More specifically, HIAA suggested that "the evaluation of the financial impact of proposed new facilities and services by the rate review authority must be considered in the certificate of need process. The effectiveness of any certificate of need agency in allocating new capital expenditures or promoting relocation, merger, and closure of facilities and services will depend in great part on the fiscal sanctions of the budget review mechanism. Therefore, in evaluating increased capital expenditures, the [state] commission should approve costs only for those services and facilities which have been approved by the appropriate planning agency."[40]

Similarly, HIAA and other witnesses noted that there was need for a mechanism to verify the "appropriateness" of volume increases, as well as the impact of revenue restraints on the quality of the care provided. It was suggested that coordination between rate or budget review and PSROs could accomplish this purpose, although PSRO review would have to be extended beyond the review of patients reimbursed under federal programs in order to do so.[41] Furthermore, supporters of state-run programs pointed out that it would be impossible to coordinate these programs if the authority for revenue constraints was solely federal.[42]

In opposition to the supporters of state initiatives, labor unions lobbied against the concept: "The AFL-CIO strongly favors a national program with uniform standards and uniform administration. We find no convincing evidence that these states have performed an effective job of controlling hospital costs. A study conducted by ICF Incorporated for the *Federation of American Hospitals* indicates that in 1974–1975...the annual increase in hospital expenditures on a per capita basis was 19.1 percent for the states with controls versus 18.7 percent for the states with no controls [emphasis added]."[43] What the AFL-CIO did not mention was that the Federation of American Hospitals is bitterly opposed to state-run cost containment programs,[44] and that data collected by others, specifically the Social Security Administration and HIAA, arrived at no such conclusions, as stated in Chapter 4. Labor representatives indicated their real concern in stating, "However, if despite our recommendations, the possibility for states to opt out remains, then state hospital cost containment programs must include all of the requirements of the federal law including the exclusion of nonsupervisory wages from the nine percent ceiling."[45]

More important, it should be noted that labor representatives had another item on their agenda which was not explicitly addressed during congressional deliberations, protecting the future of their National Health Insurance proposal—the Health Security bill. Health Security is a totally federal program and one which envisages little role for the states. Richard Shoemaker of the AFL-CIO Department of Social Security alluded to labor's agenda by reminding the senators that "the Administration indicates that they will have at least guidelines for a national health insurance program by March 31, 1978. Now, the problem in dealing with temporary programs is that you are setting—and you do not know what national health insurance program is going to be like, that you are already preempting it to a certain extent, and setting formulations which probably may be in contradiction to any program to be handed down. Now, certainly one of the big issues of national health insurance is whether the program should require a single payer, or a Federal-State program, or whatnot."[46] In a significant blow to supporters of the proposal, labor representatives later announced that because subsequent drafts broadened the options for state-run programs labor support could not be assured.

The Impact of Proponents' Efforts

Little heavy lobbying was conducted by supporters of the bill, and the lack of support by labor unions is detrimental to any legislation even though their support alone may not be enough to pass a bill. HIAA and the National Conference of State Legislatures provided valuable assistance in drafting and lobbying for the state-option bills described in the next chapter, but there was little activity in support of the entire bill.

What they, or the health planning groups, consumer groups, or other governmental groups did not do was to organize a letter-writing campaign or "haunt" the halls of Congress in an attempt to line up support for the legislation, even after it was modified, as did their colleagues in the opposition. Instead, the effort to impose some form of constraint on the hospital industry was left to HEW and to individual congressmen and their staffs who felt that the time had come to impose those restraints. The next chapter describes the response of those congressmen who found themselves in general philosophical agreement with the idea of imposing restraints, the specific modifications made in an effort to make it more palatable to both opponents and proponents, and the reaction those modifications engendered.

III | The Congressional Response

7 | The Initial Response

In contrast to the speedy response of the critics, the response of Congress had consumed over 17 months at this writing. Criticism of the general thrust of the legislation was loud and long, and pointed comments about the technical aspects of the bill were often difficult to understand. Accompanying the complexity of technical details was considerable concern that many of the legislation's provisions were inequitable or incorrectly focused, and individual congressmen set their staffs to work to design more palatable legislation. The subsequent introduction of alternative proposals, therefore, led to further compounding of the difficulties faced by Congress in passing cost containment legislation and to a further lengthening of the process. (See Table 7–1 for a comparison of the various bills.)

H.R. 8121 (Rogers)

The first congressman to respond to the administration's proposal by introducing an alternative based on the administration's bill was Paul Rogers (D.-Fla.), chairman of the Commerce Health Subcommittee. Rogers enjoys wide respect for his expertise in the health care field, and his sponsorship of many federal health care initiatives has earned him the title "Mr. Health." For this reason, his less-than-enthusiastic response to the administration's proposal, as demonstrated by his June 30, 1977 statement accompanying his new proposal, was a good indication of the prospects for passing H.R. 6575 speedily, or without substantial modification:

> Although I am not yet convinced that the approach to stemming inflation in the health care sector embodied in H.R. 6575 is entirely appropriate, I am today using it as a vehicle for three new concepts which, in my judgment deserve the consideration of Congress and other affected parties.

These new proposals are offered, not with the intent that they represent my position on cost containment, but rather, in anticipation of thorough debate on their merits, cost, and practicability. As time permits other ideas to be developed, I will submit additional legislative proposals to bring these ideas and concepts into the public domain. In my view, through this procedure, we can best assure a thorough consideration of this complicated issue.[1]

Notwithstanding Rogers' concern about the "appropriateness" of H.R. 6575, the new bill, H.R. 8121, made almost no modification to the original proposal. It retained the revenue cap, the same admission load formula, the same base year, the same exceptions process, and the $2.5 billion cap on capital expenditures. The bill did make one change to Title I, in reflection of Rogers' concern that the proposal was too much of a "stick" without any "carrot," i.e., it added a small incentive payment program for those hospitals which kept the rate of increase below the promulgated revenue limit. Under this program the hospital could receive one-third of the difference between the revenue cap and the hospital's actual rate of increase, as long as it was lower than the cap. The revenue realized by the hospital under the program could be applied only to the hospital's outpatient department deficit, and the hospital could not receive any funds *in excess* of the outpatient deficit.

The proposal would not have had a very broad effect because only 1,423 hospitals out of about 6,000 in the country had previously kept their rate of increase below the proposed 9 percent limit.[2] AHA pointed out that only 2,028 hospitals had an organized outpatient department; the number experiencing a deficit would be even less.[3]

A much broader and more important provision of H.R. 8121 was that it extended the certificate of need program beyond the institutional setting. In effect, it would extend regulation into private physician's offices which meant the possible active opposition of the AMA, although information supplied by Blue Cross indicated that the only piece of major medical equipment to be regulated under the proposed $150,000 threshold for certificate of need review would be the C.A.T. scanner.[4]

Many people have been concerned about the unchecked proliferation of expensive medical equipment in clinics and physician's offices, with the resultant impact on overall health care costs. This point of view is reflected in the Rogers bill. It is certainly a reasonable point that if physicians purchased equipment which essentially put them in competition with hospitals, they should be required to follow the same regulatory procedures as hospitals already were bound by.

The Rogers proposal also made several other changes in the certificate of need program. The proposal required the secretary of HEW to dis-

Table 7-1

Comparison of Major Provisions of Cost Containment Bills

	H.R. 6575 S. 1391 Administration	H.R. 8121 Rogers	H.R. 8337 Rostenkowski	H.R. 8687 Carter	S. 1878 Schweiker	S. 1470 (as revised) Talmadge
1. Report on Permanent Reform	x	x	x	*	*	0
2. Transitional Revenue						
Limitation	x	x	*	x	x	*
Hospital Cost Index	0	0	0	*	0	*
Exemption for Small Hospitals	0	0	*	0	0	0
3. State Plan Option	x	x	x	*	*	*
Federal Funding for State Programs	0	0	0	*	*	0
4. Capital Expenditure Control	x	x	0	x	*	0
Dollar Limits	x	x	0	x	0	0
Bed and Occupancy Limits	x	x	0	x[1]	x	0
Decertification	0	0	0	*	*	0
5. Coverage under Certificate of Need for Medical Equipment in Physician's Offices	0	*	0	0	0	0
6. Incentives for Discontinuing Services	0	*	0	*	*	*

Explanation of Symbols:

x = provision similar to administration's proposal is included in bill.
* = provision introduced in this bill differs from administration's proposal.
0 = no similar provision included in bill.
[1]H.R. 8687 does not include an occupancy standard.

allow any amount attributable to depreciation, interest, return or equity, or any other expense relating to unapproved capital expenditures, and any amount attributable to the expense of operating an unapproved facility, service, or piece of equipment. The present law only denies an amount equal to depreciation, interest, and return on equity, while H.R. 6575 required the denial of an amount equal to ten times these three factors.

Perhaps the most important change H.R. 8121 would have made to federal certificate of need requirements was that no capital expenditure would be approved in a state which did not have a program consistent with the requirements proposed by H.R. 8121. No state had a program consistent with the proposal and, therefore, the bill provided for a virtual moratorium on new capital expenditures until such time as the secretary promulgated new regulations and each state changed its laws or regulations to follow suit.

The bill would also have stiffened the planning process by requiring the sellers of medical equipment to assure that certificate of need approval had been obtained by the buyer before the sale. Failure to comply with this requirement would make the seller liable to a civil penalty not to exceed five times the price of the equipment. Another new requirement proposed by H.R. 8121 was that a certificate of need could not have been approved by a state, except in cases of emergency, unless the capital expenditure involved was previously included in the institution's capital plan submitted to the local health planning agency.

The Rogers proposal also contained another set of incentives designed to assist and encourage the discontinuance of unneeded hospital services, a radical departure from H.R. 6575. The new Title III added by H.R. 8121 to the cost containment bills directs the secretary to establish guidelines for each health service and for the "minimum appropriate use" of those services. The health systems agencies would be directed to use these guidelines to identify the actions necessary to bring the HSA into compliance, and would review applications by hospitals for discontinuance or conversion of those services and facilities deemed to be unneeded. The State Health Planning and Development Agency would review the applications with the recommendations of the HSA, and forward them to the secretary for review. The secretary was required to give priority to the applications which resulted in the greatest reduction in hospital revenues within a health service area.

Each hospital whose application was approved would be eligible for an incentive payment for closure or conversion. In the case of total closure, the payment would equal the hospital's outstanding debt less the fair market value of the hospital's assets plus an incentive payment equal to 5 percent of the hospital's revenue or $500,000, whichever was less. Hospitals closing identifiable service units, but not the whole hospital, could receive a smaller incentive payment but not a debt payment. Last, hospitals which converted unneeded beds or facilities into either long-term care or outpatient facilities could receive an incentive payment of up to 50 percent of the costs of conversion.

Although the payment was termed a "voluntary" program for the close-out of excess capacity, it did contain a penalty if the health service area did not meet the guidelines within the four-year period of the program. The penalty would have reduced by 5 percent the federal reimbursement to each hospital deemed unneeded in whole or in part by the HSA if the standards were not met.

The Subcommittee on Health and the Environment held hearings on H.R. 8121 on July 18, 1977, although most of the short list of witnesses reiterated their stand on H.R. 6575. HEW stated that H.R. 6575 already contained enough incentives to save money and that a specific payment program was unnecessary.[5] AHA was supportive, noting that it thought that incentives were a good idea, but explained that the scope of the program should be broadened.[6]

Not surprisingly, AMA came out strongly against the extension of certificate of need, and also stated that a program designed to reduce excess capacity would result "in a lowering of quality of care available to all citizens."[7] HEW also did not support the excess capacity reduction program, noting, "We do not believe that such detailed provisions can be put into place in the context of the transitional legislation which is being considered by the Committee at this time. We believe that it would be more appropriate for these sorts of programs to be developed and included as part of legislation, such as the amendments to the planning act or national health insurance, which will be considered by the committee in the coming months."[8]

This is an interesting statement, and a further consideration of its background provides insight into why the administration has had difficulty in passing the hospital cost containment bill. The H.R. 8121 Title III proposal had been developed by a member of Rogers' staff, and was circulated in draft form to interested parties as early as May 1977. It was clearly a congressional initiative. The curious point is that the administration's proposed health planning amendments introduced in March 1978 contained a close-out program very similar to that proposed officially by Rogers in June 1977. At that time the administration supported it wholeheartedly. However, HEW at least raises suspicions when it claims that what it could not do in June 1977, it can do in March 1978. The impression left in the minds of congressmen is that HEW would not support anything that it did not think of first, a position which obviously does not sit well with decision makers on Capitol Hill. In HEW's defense, it did not vigorously fight the inclusion of the program in the cost containment bill and, in fact, developed the data necessary to defend it.

The important point about H.R. 8121 is that the three proposals contained within it did not substantially modify the thrust of the administration's proposal, and the reaction to the bill was therefore somewhat muted. As noted by Rogers, the bill did not represent his last words on the subject, and he was later to propose significant amendments to the administration's proposed Hospital Cost Containment Act (H.R. 6575) during his subcommittee's mark-up of the bill. The other major bills introduced on cost containment proposed much more significant changes in the administration's bill, as members sought to find a more agreeable solution to the problem.

H.R. 8337 (Rostenkowski)

Mr. Rostenkowski (D.-Ill.), chairman of the Subcommittee on Health of the Committee on Ways and Means, introduced his proposed revisions (H.R. 8337) to the administration's proposal on July 14, 1977. The bill was cosponsored by five of the seven Democratic members of his subcommittee. In his remarks at the time of introduction of the amendments, Rostenkowski noted, "Public hearings on the administration's proposal. . . produced a variety of detailed comment and criticism. I have directed the staff of the Subcommittee, based on their study of these comments and others, to consider what options might be available to respond to the most significant criticisms of the Administration's bill. I am today introducing legislation which offers alternatives to several of the most highly criticized features of the Administration's bill. These changes are designed to preserve the intent of the Administration's bill while improving its workability and acceptability."[9]

The first change proposed by Rostenkowski in response to the criticisms leveled at H.R. 6575 was to put a four-year limit on the transitional program. As an approach directed at solving the retroactivity problem raised by AHA, H.R. 8337 applies the revenue cap to hospital fiscal reporting periods beginning after December 31, 1977.

In a significant departure from the administration, Rostenkowski proposed that the revenue limit equal a flat 9 percent which did not diminish over time as did the revenue limit in the administration's proposal. Unfortunately, from the hospitals' point of view, the 9 percent limit would be applied in an additive manner to revenue calculated from the base year. Therefore, the actual allowable percentage increase over the previous accounting year would decrease to about 7 percent in the fourth year of the program. Also, since the cap was not in any way related to the rate of inflation in the economy, the hospitals might end up in a tight squeeze if the prevailing rate of inflation rose, as it would, for example, if Congress ever passed the energy bill.

The Rostenkowski bill also deleted the provision in H.R. 6575 that no revenue increase would be provided for admission increases of less than 2 percent. As a result, the revenue limit would be raised at a rate equal to one-half the average per admission payment for each additional admission over the base year.

In an effort to answer the charge that the administration's proposal (H.R. 6575) unfairly penalized those hospitals which had worked to become efficient while rewarding inefficient hospitals, the Rostenkowski bill (H.R. 8337) contained an incentive adjustment based upon the grouping methodology contained in Section 223 of P.L. 92-603. A hospital below the median would be permitted to increase its revenue cap up to the median level, but in no case by more than one-fourth. Similarly, hospitals above the median for their group could have their revenue limit reduced toward the median but, again, by no more than one-fourth.

Exceptions to the revenue limit would have been granted under H.R. 8337 much as they would be under H.R. 6575, but special provision for granting an exception was made in H.R. 8337 when an increase in in-patient insurance coverage caused a hospital's revenues to increase by more than 3 percent, or when variations in the source of reimbursement caused revenues to decrease by 3 percent or more. H.R. 8337 also removed the requirement that hospitals be in the lowest quartile of all hospitals in regard to the institutions' current ratio before exceptions could be granted. Hospitals would have to meet only the requirement that some unusual circumstance had occurred, such as a large increase in admissions, and the revenue limit would be increased to the extent necessary to restore the current ratio to the same level as existed in the hospital's base year.

In another key change to the administration's proposal, Rostenkowski proposed that approximately 3,200 small hospitals with fewer than 4,000 annual admissions be exempted entirely from the program. The administration's proposal provided these hospitals only with a more liberal volume load adjustment in consideration of the fact that a smaller hospital has fewer patients over which to spread fixed costs, and small changes in admissions cause fixed costs per patient to vary widely. In opposition to the proposal HEW claimed that "it is our experience that the percentage increase in hospital costs did not differ by type of hospital. If you are looking at levels, that is a different matter, but if you're talking about a percentage increase, that doesn't vary between large and small."[10] Data supplied by HEW, however, show this statement to be questionable in that small hospital costs increased 1.2 percent faster than large ones in 1976.[11] Moreover, these small hospitals constitute about one-half of all the hospitals in the United States, and they consume only about 13 percent of total hospital expenditures.[12] Exempting them from the program represented a large simplification and, therefore, constituted a plausible change for many congressmen, not to mention that it would remove a significant amount of local pressure in opposition to the bill. Rostenkowski further improved the plausability of his proposal by requiring the small hospitals to publish any cost or charge increase which was in excess of the revenue limit, thereby providing some protection to patients who were served by those hospitals.

Rostenkowski also proposed that one of the barriers to state cost containment programs be removed from the administration's cost containment bill. As opposed to the administration's proposed requirement that state programs meet the promulgated revenue limit, H.R. 8337 provided that the allowable revenue limit for state programs could include consideration of not only the amount of the promulgated federal revenue limit, but also the amount of wage pass-throughs and exceptions granted.

Rostenkowski did not propose to remove the requirements that state programs be in operation for one year, cover 90 percent of the hospitals in the state, and cover all non-Medicare payers immediately, nor did he propose to provide any incentives to state governments to institute a program. The further encouragement of state cost containment programs was left to the next two major proposals to be discussed.

S. 1878 (Schweiker) and H.R. 8687 (Carter)

On July 15, 1977, Representative Tim Lee Carter (R.-Ky.), ranking minority member of the Rogers subcommittee, announced his intention to introduce a new cost containment proposal, noting, "Although I share the Administration's desire for timely action to remedy the problem of rapidly escalating hospital costs, I feel that the Administration's proposal is not properly focused, nor can it accomplish the long-term goals toward which we should be working."[13]

One of Carter's major concerns was that hospitals vary widely in terms of size, location, services, case mix, and efficiency, and, therefore, he did not believe it either feasible or desirable to institute a program solely at the federal level. Instead, Carter proposed that the states be the focus of the cost containment program:

I submit that only a program instituted at the state level...can achieve the level of specificity and sophistication necessary to insure that desired efficiency is achieved while maintaining quality of care. Such a program must insure that needed facilities are not forced to close; it must insure that base year budgets are "reasonable" and it must insure that utilization levels represent care which is needed. This is a complex and difficult task and cannot be accomplished by the imposition of a simple formula, as proposed by the Administration. More importantly, an effective budget review system must be linked to the planning and utilization review systems if it is to insure support for needed, effective, efficient health care institutions. The Federal Government has already instituted planning programs under Public Law 93-641, and utilization review and quality assurance programs under Public Law 92-603, which are based at the state and local level. It is difficult to see how these activities could be effectively linked to the cost containment program if it were based in Washington.[14]

In the Senate, Senator Richard Schweiker, ranking minority member of the Kennedy subcommittee, and his staff were working on a similar proposal; Schweiker had announced his intention to introduce an alternative proposal in a statement to the Senate two weeks before:

I am announcing today my intentions to introduce legislation emphasizing State control of costs as an alternative to the...short-sighted stop-gap measure [proposed by the administration].

One of the most pressing issues facing this nation today is the skyrocketing cost of health care. But contrary to President Carter, I believe that we must get the States to attack this problem rather than use an already bloated Federal bureaucracy to impose purely Federal controls. State and local officials are more in tune with the unique health care needs of their communities and with the specific steps which would be most effective in curbing sharply rising health care costs.[15]

Schweiker's bill, S. 1878, was introduced July 18, 1977 and Carter's bill, H.R. 8687, was introduced August 2, 1977. Since H.R. 8687 contained much of the same language as did S. 1878, the prevailing wisdom at the time was that Schweiker had provided the impetus for the Carter bill. Such was not the case; rather, it was a situation in which two different sets of people working with similar information arrived at similar conclusions. Both staffs had been provided with a copy of a Government Research Corporation report on a proposal for state rate setting.[16] Schweiker recently had hired a new staff person fresh from the government of the state of California, while Carter had just hired a new staff person who recently had participated in a study on the linkage among rate review, planning, and utilization review for the Subcommittee on Oversight and Investigations. Also, Schweiker's staff were being advised by a professor from Yale University's Department of Epidemiology and Public Health under whom Carter's new staff member had recently completed a course of study.

Perhaps the most interesting thing about the Carter/Schweiker proposals was that they were even made at all, regardless of the similar points of view represented in the respective staffs. Both men have a reputation as conservative Republicans, who are not known for their philosophic support of greater federal regulation, and both bills envisioned a modified federal transitional program which would yield to state programs after they were established.

Representative Carter is a physician from a rural area in Kentucky which continues to experience significant poverty. As demonstrated by the recent strike by the United Mine Workers, one of the major concerns of Carter's constituents is the cost of health care, a major point of contention in that strike. Nonetheless, Carter maintains close ties with the AMA, and has expressed on countless occasions his fear that any restraints on health care resources will interfere with high quality health care. Against that fear, however, is a significant concern for the welfare of the people in his district. It is interesting to note in this regard that Carter's office made more inquiries in 1977 to the Social Security Administration than did any other congressional office, including Senate offices.[17] The important point for Dr. Carter, then, was to balance these two interests; the provision in his bill which brings local physicians, through the PSROs, and other community leaders, through the HSAs, into the process was his way of doing it. Political reality also played a role in that the Democrats have a two-to-one edge over the Republicans in the House. Dr. Carter expressed the view that the best way to get some of what you want is to compromise with the majority while doing all that you can to improve the proposed legislation.[18]

Specifically, these two minority members (Carter and Schweiker) proposed that the whole focus of the transitional program be changed so that it would operate only in those states that did not have an approved state cost containment program, with federal funding made available to assist states in instituting a program. Both bills required the institution of state commissions which would review budgets prospectively, although the Schweiker bill required the commission to approve rates, while the Carter bill focused on the approval of budgets. Also, both bills specifically required the state commissions to allow hospitals to retain any surplus they were able to generate through keeping spending levels below the approved rate.

Both bills restricted the power of the federal government to preempt state programs to those states which could not maintain an aggregate rate of increase less than or equal to the federal program, with the Carter bill making it clear that the allowable rate was the promulgated revenue increase limit *plus* any adjustments and exceptions. The Carter bill exempted state programs from any permanent program as well.

The process of linking the PSROs and health planning to rate or budget review was reflected in the Schweiker bill by giving the state commission the power to review any capital expenditures which would have an impact upon hospital rates. The bill also extended PSRO review to all classes of patients (PSRO review presently only applies to federally reimbursed patients) and provided that the cost of such a review would be included in the hospital's approved rates.

In reflection of Carter's concern on this point, his bill contained a more explicit set of linkage mechanisms. Under H.R. 8687, health planning agencies and state budget review commissions would be required to enter into a formal memorandum of agreement concerning data sharing, development of complementary guidelines and procedures for review, and coordinated activities in reference to state health plans. State budget commissions would also be required to review the financial feasibility of all certificate of need applications, although the final determination of need would remain with the state-level health planning agencies and the local health systems agencies. Carter's bill also provided for an extension of PSRO review to all classes of patients, and for memoranda of agreement between the PSROs and the state budget commissions regarding data sharing and joint development of quality assurance systems. Perhaps the Carter bill's most significant departure from the Schweiker proposal was its stipulation that the state's exemption from the federal program, and the federal designation of the state-level health planning agencies and of the PSROs, be contingent upon their entering into the required cooperative agreements.

The Schweiker bill made no significant changes in the transitional program which would operate while the states were setting up their programs. Carter proposed changes which reflected some of the concerns raised by witnesses at the hearings. H.R. 8687 would have brought the base year forward to fiscal reporting periods ending after September 30, 1976, as a means of reducing the inequities associated with a base year set too far in the past. Carter also proposed that the secretary develop a new index of hospital input costs so that the argument consistently raised by AHA about the role of cost-push inflation could finally be put to rest, and wage increases could be recognized without a pass-through.

An important proposal of Carter's, which was to gain widespread acceptance, was a provision designed to turn around one of the backwards incentives caused by the admission load formula contained in the administration's proposal (H.R. 6575). The administration's admission load formula was included to discourage additional hospital admissions. Unfortunately, it might also discourage the sharing of medical service units because the hospital providing the service would not have received full reimbursement for the extra admissions which a shared-service arrangement might cause. Carter's bill remedied this problem, stating that the additional admissions caused by the shared-service arrangement would be added to the hospital's base year volume, thus insuring that full reimbursement would be received. For a hospital losing a service, H.R. 6575 (administration) had provided that a hospital would not incur any loss in revenue if the service was found to be unneeded by a health planning agency; H.R. 8687 (Carter) treated hospitals which lost volume as a result of a shared-service agreement in a similar fashion.

In further recognition of the importance of reducing excess capacity, both the Schweiker and Carter bills raised a trial balloon on the subject of decertification. With identical language the bills proposed that state-level planning agencies be empowered to declare certain health care facilities and services as surplus. Facilities and services so declared would then be considered for federal reimbursement purposes as if they had never received a certificate of need; therefore, they would become ineligible for federal reimbursement. As if to remove the sting of that provision, the bills authorized payment of grants to institutions in need of funds to retire the outstanding indebtedness of the facility or a service declared as surplus.

Finally, the two bills (H.R. 8687 and S. 1878) proposed different changes to the administration's capital expenditure limitations. With some exceptions, Schweiker proposed a flat moratorium on hospital capital expenditures for 18 months. This provision was included to allow state-level health planning agencies time to become established and to implement the decertification provisions contained in the bill. In consideration of Congressman Carter's concern about the effects of such a moratorium on needed quality health care, H.R. 8687 did not go that far. Carter accepted the administration's basic $2.5 billion capital expenditure limitation but proposed that it be allocated among the states on the basis of the ratio of the historical cost (minus accumulated depreciation) of hospital assets to the population of the state. This allocation measure was intended to provide a rough estimate of the need for capital expenditures since the ratio would take into account the relative value and the relative age of hospitals in a state. Carter also proposed that 20 percent of the total limit be held in reserve by the secretary to be allocated to national health resource centers (such as the Mayo Clinic, the Cleveland Clinic, and others), and to states which the secretary determined to have significant unmet health needs.

Both of these proposals were referred to the respective Senate and

House subcommittees and were considered along with the proposals of the majority members. The bills were an important part of the congressional response to the administration's proposal as they put the ranking minority members of two of the four subcommittees working on H.R. 6575 on record as supporting its basic thrust, and that support was valuable to the proponents of the original proposal. Although the Schweiker and Carter bills soon disappeared as discrete pieces of legislation, many of their provisions, as well as those of H.R. 8121 and H.R. 8337, were to appear in subsequent drafts of the administration's bill. In contrast, the final proposal to be discussed does not appear in any draft of the administration's proposal, nor was it formally considered by three of the four subcommittees; it is a radically different proposal from that of the administration.

S. 1470 (Talmadge)

S. 1470 was introduced on May 5, 1977 by Senator Herman Talmadge (D.-Ga.), chairman of the Subcommittee on Health of the Committee on Finance. It was a similar proposal to a bill (S. 3205) introduced by Talmadge in the previous Congress. As originally introduced, S. 1470 did not focus on cost containment per se, but proposed reforms in the way reasonable costs were determined for Medicare and Medicaid reimbursement. For that reason, Talmadge claimed that the two proposals were not in conflict: "My proposal represents a long-term basic structural answer to the problem of rising hospital costs, whereas the Administration is calling for a short-term interim cap on revenues to be in place only until a long-term solution can be established."[19] Talmadge also indicated that the long-term approach which he envisioned would be that embodied in S. 1470, although he was less certain of his final conclusion about the merits of the administration's proposal as an interim cap.

Specifically, S. 1470 proposed that all hospitals be classified and categorized according to size, type, and other criteria which the secretary might find appropriate; in addition, an average per diem routine operating cost would be determined for each group. Medicare and Medicaid reimbursement payments would then be based upon these group averages; there would be incentive payments for lower than average cost hospitals, and reduced payments for higher cost hospitals. Adjustments and special allowances would be provided based upon price increases, location in a medical shortage area, and other "appropriate factors."

Although the Talmadge bill did not originally contain any revenue increase limits other than limiting hospitals to average routine costs, it did reflect some of the concerns raised in other forums, i.e., exemptions for state programs, incentives for closure or conversion, disallowance of direct operating costs caused by unapproved capital expenditures, and provisions to remove inconsistencies between the National Health Planning and Resources Development Act of 1974 and Section 1122 of the Social Security Act.

One problem with the Talmadge bill was that although it contained the first attempt to break the existing connection between hospitals' cost increases and automatic revenue increases, it did not go far enough. First, the new reimbursement system envisioned by the bill would not go into effect until 1981. Second, the bill only applied its controls to the portion of routine operating cost reimbursable by Medicare and Medicaid. As a result, all ancillary costs were excluded as well as capital costs, education costs, energy costs, and malpractice insurance costs. The limited application of the proposed system meant that in the first year the program was to be implemented (1981), total savings estimates ranged only from $100 million to $400 million.

A further problem was that although the bill incorporated many of the sophisticated concepts developed in state rate review programs or proposed in the literature (e.g., grouping, uniform accounting, positive and negative incentives, and adjustment of the reimbursement system to pay for closure or convention), some of these concepts were used in what seemed to be a loose and somewhat ill-defined fashion. For example, the grouping methodology included only 4 basic variables (size, short-term general hospitals, teaching, and other specialty hospitals); in contrast the Washington State program bases its grouping system on 18 variables. In applying the reimbursement limits, S. 1470 (Talmadge) proposed that hospitals be allowed up to 120 percent of the average group costs, a relatively wide corridor. This is not to say that the grouping system or the payment corridor envisioned by S. 1470 could not be used at a later time; the immediate problem was that S. 1470's system was not operationally defensible and Talmadge was proposing to lock the basic thrust of the system into the federal statute, although the system did provide for adjustments as it was implemented.

The problems associated with the methodology of S. 1470 were subordinated to Senator Talmadge's continued strong support for his proposal. Hindsight indicates that the senator did very little to move the administration's proposal forward. Instead of holding hearings on the administration's bill, Talmadge held hearings on his own and continued his lack of movement on S. 1391 (administration proposal) throughout the summer of 1977. His recalcitrance led the president to write a letter to the senator, informing him of the president's "strong personal commitment to the Administration's Hospital Cost Containment Legislation.''[20] The same day the president wrote to Senator Kennedy praising him for his efforts in behalf of the administration's proposal.[21]

Bowing somewhat to the pressure, Talmadge put his staff to work revising his proposal so that it would be effective July 1, 1978, cover all payers, and include ancillary costs. The new proposal, released as a working draft in early October 1977, applied a routine revenue limitation based upon group averages to hospital routine costs on a per diem basis. Borrowing from the administration's proposal, the new draft further envisioned the application of an ancillary revenue limitation on a per admission basis. The ancillary revenue limitation was a flat percentage cap applied to the previous year's ancillary revenue, and was to be based upon prevailing wage rates in the hospital's locality and on a national index devised by the HEW secretary's which measured changes in the hospital "market basket."

Talmadge's subcommittee finally held hearings on cost containment beginning October 12, 1977, although most of the comments were directed toward the Talmadge proposal rather than the administration's bill. Most witnesses indicated their general approval of Talmadge's efforts to recognize regional differences, input prices, and the need for positive incentives. Criticism was directed toward the sensitivity of the grouping system, and the inclusion of a flat cap for ancillary services. The comment made most often by witnesses representing provider groups was that they preferred any Talmadge-like proposal to the legislation proposed by the administration.

Nevertheless, the three other subcommittees under whose jurisdiction the cost containment bill fell were moving ahead with legislation substantially similar to the administration's proposal. Talmadge's subcommittee, in contrast, took no further action on either of the two proposals before it. This approach effectively kept any cost containment proposal from reaching the floor of the Senate regardless of what Senator Kennedy's subcommittee did. Moreover, Talmadge's inaction during a period in which all of the other subcommittees began to move forward on cost containment put the senator in a key position to extract concessions from the administration on the shape of a cost containment program, although in the muddled situation existing on this issue the dimensions of those concessions were something at which observers could only guess.

Conclusion

One important point which was clear at this point in the legislative process was that the administration was not going to get the speedy enactment of cost containment legislation for which it had hoped. Senator Talmadge did not schedule hearings until after the program start-up date included in the administration's bill. Moreover, even in the three subcommittees which tried to move ahead with the proposal in a reasonably expeditious fashion, there were now several different proposals to consider. It should also be remembered that only the chairmen and the ranking minority members of the subcommittees had staff working full-time on analyzing the various proposals; therefore, all of the various methods of administering the program embodied in the different bills, and all of the estimated effects of the program had to be explained to other subcommittee members and to their staffs.

Overlying this technical complexity was a general uneasiness and concern with the effects of the cost containment bills on the production of needed health care services, and the efforts of lobbyists to amplify those concerns. In consideration of these factors, few on Capitol Hill were expecting quick resolution of the cost containment question, although no observers expected it to take as long as it did.

Three of the four subcommittees attempted to move forward with the legislation during the summer and fall of 1977, and two were actually able to report a bill to their respective full committees. The next chapter describes those efforts.

8 | Progress

Procedural Note

After the information gathering phase represented by hearings and staff discussions, the usual next step in the approval of a bill is a subcommittee mark-up, although this step can be skipped. During a mark-up the subcommittee staff presents the legislation and provides the members with information on each provision as well as describing any alternatives which may exist. Subcommittee members may also present formal admendments at this and subsequent points in the process. Many of the decisions regarding the shape of the legislation may have been negotiated in advance of the public mark-up sessions and, therefore, the mark-up itself may only be a *pro forma* discussion of decisions already made. Each subcommittee has a different way of proceeding depending upon the policies of the chairman, the relationships among the members (especially between majority and minority), the general level of interest of the members in the issue at hand, and other factors. However the subcommittee reaches agreement, whether through prior negotiation, discussion, debate, formal votes, or a combination of these methods, its basic task is to agree on the legislation and to report the subcommittee's version to its parent full committee. The full committee follows a similar process in reporting a bill to the floor of the House or Senate.

Unfortunately from a historical viewpoint, generally no record of the mark-up sessions is kept; therefore, a report of the proceedings must rely upon the legislation actually reported, and the memories of observers.

For that reason, the account presented below is quite complete in regard to the deliberations of the Commerce Subcommittee on Health and the Environment, in which the senior author participated, but is somewhat limited regarding the other subcommittees concerned.

The First Step: Committee on Human Resources

The first subcommittee to take action on the cost containment bill was Senator Kennedy's Subcommittee on Health and Scientific Research. The subcommittee met briefly to consider both the administration's proposal and the bill introduced by Senator Schweiker. Without formal action on either, it referred the process of mark-up to the full Senate Human Resources Committee on July 25, 1977. Before the subcommittee met, however, Kennedy's staff had developed a bill which made several significant changes to the administration's proposal, and the staff also had engaged in a process of negotiation with Senator Schweiker's staff regarding the minority's concerns.

According to a member of the minority staff, these negotiations revolved around two basic issues, state exemptions and the wage pass-through.[1] Consistent with organized labor's point of view, Kennedy's staff argued that there were no state rate review programs which had shown an ability to constrain costs. With information and assistance provided by the Health Insurance Association of America and by the American Hospital Association, Schweiker's staff argued the opposite. The argument over the wage pass-through followed similar lines with the majority arguing for the mandatory pass-through favored by labor and the minority arguing against it, as favored by HIAA and AHA.

Presumably as a result of prior negotiation, the committee mark-up sessions were brief. Except for the question of an exemption for small hospitals, the only issues discussed were the two on which the staff had not been able to reach agreement. These issues were the state exemption and the wage pass-through, with the pass-through being the more troublesome.

The resulting bill reflected many of the concerns raised during hearings and in staff discussions, but it did not go as far in revising the administration's proposal as would other versions. The committee draft continued the use of a revenue limit formula based on the GNP deflator, although, as in H.R. 8687 (Carter), HEW would be directed to develop an index which "more accurately reflects the rate of increase in the prices of inputs necessary for the production and delivery of hospital services."[2] The draft did not contain a termination date as in the Rosten-kowski bill (H.R. 8337). However, it did apply the revenue limit to the previous year's revenue, rather than to a base year, thereby reducing the double ratchet effect against which AHA had fought so hard. In a fashion somewhat similar to the Rogers bill (H.R. 8121), the committee draft provided for exceptions based upon changes in benefits, reimbursement methodology, and patient mix among payers. The committee also decided to exempt small hospitals.

The most significant departures from the administration's proposal occurred in the areas of the wage pass-through, exemptions for state programs, the admission load formula, and capital expenditure limitations. First, the committee honored labor's wishes by making the wage pass-through mandatory; the hospital would have to split its cost into labor and nonlabor components, with the revenue increase limit applying only to that percentage of costs attributable to nonlabor items. The bill proposed that the actual increase in labor costs would be added to the resultant nonlabor figure to arrive at a total revenue limit.

As a result of the efforts of Schweiker and his staff, the committee draft significantly expanded opportunities for states to operate their own programs. A variety of payment control mechanisms would be permitted, as long as the states gave assurance that the aggregate rate of increase under their programs would not be less than the GNP deflator nor more than 110 percent of the promulgated revenue increase limit. In outlining the general shape of federal government requirements for state programs, the committee picked up much of the language from Schweiker's bill (S. 1878) and authorized $10 million for support of the state initiatives.

The committee departed from Schweiker's state plan in a curious way by stipulating that the wage pass-through was to be made mandatory for state programs, except in the estimated seven states with existing programs which would have qualified immediately for an exemption. The mandatory nature of the pass-through was the most objectionable provision of the bill for the minority members of the committee, and led to the filing of minority views in the committee report on behalf of Senators Schweiker, Hatch, and Hayakawa. The minority termed the provision "inequitable," and pointed out that the available evidence did not support the need for the pass-through:

> The faster than average wage increases received by hospital workers in recent years have done much to eliminate past disparities....
> The available data do not support the contention that nonsupervisory hospital employees, *as a group,* are systematically underpaid relative to the wage-levels of their nonhospital peers. They reveal instead a patchwork pattern of varying wage levels, within which some nonsupervisory hospital workers are underpaid and some are overpaid relative to the going rate,

depending on their geographic area and particular occupation within the hospital community. These facts hardly justify a sweeping nationwide exemption for all nonsupervisory workers' wage increases, particularly when balanced against the damage such a provision would cause the cost containment effort.[3]

It is difficult to appreciate the majority's justification for an uneven application of the pass-through to states, in light of the data from which the minority was working. Moreover, the minority repeatedly pointed out that the whole reason it was supporting state efforts was its belief that the states could devise specific, sophisticated control methodologies which could directly deal with the problem of nonsupervisory wages, thereby making blanket pass-throughs of any kind unnecessary. Nonetheless, elegant reasoning and explicit data were less important in this case than the powerful labor lobby which opposed the minority's point of view; therefore, the minority's argument did not prevail.

The minority had greater success in promoting another provision of Schweiker's bill, the capital expenditure moratorium, since its views coincided with the views of Kennedy and the majority staff. The committee draft provided for a temporary 18-month moratorium, with few exceptions, on capital expenditures exceeding $150,000 by *any* individual, including physicians, engaged in the delivery of health services. Individual states could escape the moratorium if they had an approved State Health Planning and Development Agency that administered a certificate of need program under the National Health Planning and Resources Development Act or under Section 1122 of the Social Security Act. In addition, the state must have completed action on a State Medical Facilities Plan required by the second title of the health planning act.

An interesting aspect of the Senate Human Resources Committee's plan for limiting capital expenditures was that it was very similar to the Rogers bill (H.R. 8121) and reflected the desire on the part of the health subcommittees to quicken the pace at which the states implemented the provisions of the National Health Planning and Resources Development Act. The difference between the two proposals was that the Human Resources Committee was willing to make the moratorium explicit and debate it directly on its merits. In contrast, the Rogers proposal never mentioned a moratorium, although both bills would have had the same general effect.

The most radical provision of the Human Resources bill was inclusion of Schweiker's decertification proposal, a rather startling idea in light of the furor that was later to erupt over the bed and occupancy standards proposed by the National Health Planning Guidelines discussed in

Chapter 4. Under the Human Resources proposal, Health Systems Agencies and State Health Planning and Development Agencies would continue to review the appropriateness of health facilities based upon applicable standards of need and access including those found in the national guidelines as is presently required under the National Health Planning and Resources Development Act (P.L. 93-641). In addition, Human Resources proposed that institutions and facilities found to be unneeded would be considered as if they had been denied a certificate of need, an action which would effectively cut off all federal reimbursement to such institutions or facilities.

The committee also decided to modify the admission load formula through construction of a "volume adjustment" based upon an *average* of: (1) the change in admissions and (2) the change in patient days. However, concern was expressed that the adjustment might drive costs up, given the evidence on the effect of per diem controls on volume increases. The committee also deleted the administration's provision for different corridors for different hospitals based upon their size.

The committee ordered its version of the bill reported to the floor of the Senate on August 2, 1977 on an 11 to 3 vote with Senators Schweiker, Chaffee, and Hatch casting negative votes. At this point, however, no further action could be taken in the Senate until Talmadge's subcommittee and the full Committee on Finance also reported the bill, and at this time Talmadge had not scheduled hearings on the bill. Instead, action shifted to the House of Representatives as the two House subcommittees began their attempt to get the bill passed.

The Subcommittee on Health of the Committee on Ways and Means

In late July of 1977, Congressman Rostenkowski's subcommittee began its preliminary consideration of H.R. 6575 (administration) and H.R. 8337 (Rostenkowski). Because of the press of other legislation, particularly the energy bill and the Social Security bill, the subcommittee had difficulty getting enough members to attend and was able to obtain a quorum only on July 27, 28, and 29. The subcommittee met again after the congressional recess in August in an attempt to move the bill, but was never again able to obtain a quorum.

Early in the subcommittee sessions certain trends developed which were later to have tremendous impact on the shape of the legislation and the congressional response to it. First, subcommittee members were unimpressed with the presentation of H.R. 6575 (administration) by HEW spokesmen; on occasion members were moved to laughter during the presentation. Second, tentative votes taken during the deliberations were divided along party lines with Congressmen Burleson and Pike voting with the Republican minority.[4] Thus, votes taken on two amendments offered by Republican Congressman Gradison (Ohio) to terminate the program after two years and to move the base year forward were defeated on a tie vote and a 7 to 6 vote, respectively. Although no final decisions were taken by the subcommittee before the end of the first session of the 95th Congress in December, the difficulty experienced by the subcommittee in obtaining a quorum and the division among the members on the cost containment issue led Chairman Rostenkowski to propose a radical departure from the administration's proposal. Before this was to occur, however, the other subcommittee, with jurisdiction over the legislation, the Commerce Health Subcommittee, scheduled its mark-up sessions on the bill, thereby giving the administration another chance to get its bill approved in a form similar to the one in which it had been proposed.

The Subcommittee on Health and the Environment of the Committee on Interstate and Foreign Commerce

A Question of Style

In the 95th Congress, the Subcommittee on Health and the Environment was much different from its counterpart in the Senate, the Human Resources Health Subcommittee. While the Senate subcommittee was dominated by northerners with a liberal outlook like Kennedy and Javits, the senior members of the Commerce Health Subcommittee were all southerners and more conservative. The top three on the majority side (Rogers, Satterfield, and Preyer) are from Florida, Virginia, and North Carolina respectively; while the top two on the minority side, Carter and Broyhill, are from Kentucky and North Carolina. With the exception of Waxman of California, the rest of the majority members were from the northeast. The effect of this was that when a split occurred in the subcommittee, it most often occurred between the senior members, both Republican and Democrat, and the junior Democrats. Moreover, the member who always sat on Chairman Rogers' right, Satterfield, is more conservative than Carter, who sat on the chairman's immediate left. Also, Broyhill appears to be more conservative than Carter when it comes to health issues and has stronger ties to the American Hospital Association. A recent issue of *Hospitals,* AHA's national magazine, includes an interview with Broyhill in which it appears that the Congressman's position on cost containment is very similar to that of AHA.[5]

These relationships were especially important to the issue of hospital cost containment because they meant that it was easier for Rogers and Carter to work together than it often was for either of them to work with their colleagues on their own sides of the aisle. Similarly, in consideration of the general unease expressed by many members about the cost containment bill, it was of value to Chairman Rogers to concede some points to Carter if that meant the bill would receive bipartisan support when it was reported out of the subcommittee.

Another important point which was certainly responsible for the rather consistent cooperation between Rogers and Carter is the general style in which Chairman Rogers conducts the business of his subcommittee. Rogers appears as a consensus builder who generally does not attempt to "steamroll" over those who disagree with his point of view. Carter's bill represented a distinct expression of how a hospital cost containment program should be conducted and, therefore, Rogers was receptive to incorporating that point of view into the legislation reported by the subcommittee.

When disagreement did occur, whether between Rogers and Carter or between Rogers and other Democrats, Rogers seldom called for a vote and, therefore, did not force his point of view. The more common way of proceeding was that a discussion would ensue, with Rogers attempting to find a reasonable compromise by asking the members what they thought of the idea, or whether they felt a particular approach was a reasonable way of proceeding. At this point the chairman would often turn to the HEW representatives present, normally Deputy Assistant Secretary Karen Davis or Robert O'Connor of the Health Care Financing Administration, and ask them for their opinion. In the cases in which Rogers was defending the administration's bill, the HEW people would agree with him; in other cases, HEW tended to point out why its original proposal was best. After sketching out the policy resulting from the discussion, the chairman would turn to the other members and suggest that the staff work on the issue and develop legislative language for the members to review and discuss on the following day.

The result of proceeding in such a fashion is that the subcommittee went over the entire bill three times, taking over a month to do so. The bill went through six different drafts, with both the majority and minority staff putting in long hours discussing, debating, and negotiating the specific shape of the agreements reached in the subcommittee's discussion. The most important benefit imparted by the Rogers style was that the bill produced by the subcommittee incorporated the views of most of the members and, therefore, was reported to the full Committee on Interstate and Foreign Commerce with all but three of the members

(Satterfield and two Republicans, Broyhill and Madigan) on record in support of the bill.

Preparing for Mark-Up

Before the Subcommittee on Health and the Environment began its mark-up of the cost containment bill on September 12, 1977, a great deal of time and effort had gone into analyzing the legislation and various proposed alternatives. Much discussion had occurred among HEW staff, congressional staff, and lobbyists, with each pushing a point of view, checking on the reaction to an alternative proposal, or attempting to reach a compromise.

The net result of six months of these staff-level activities was that the general shape of the legislation could have been estimated before the mark-up actually began. For example, the majority staff invited Carter's minority staff to supply what was to become a fairly vigorous defense of the policy proposed by Carter's bill for incorporation in the subcommittee briefing book prepared for members' use during the mark-up; this appeared as a good indication of the receptiveness of Chairman Rogers to the Carter proposal. More importantly, the majority staff had spent the period of preparation in devising a series of changes to the administration's proposal, and had shared it with other staff members. This provided staff members with an opportunity to discuss the proposed legislation with their congressmen and obtain their reactions to the proposals. It was possible, therefore, to ascertain on an informal basis how the subcommittee would react to a specific provision and, if necessary, to work out a compromise proposal in advance, to elicit a response from HEW and the special interest organizations, and to present it to the congressmen for their reaction. This process led to the legislation presented to the subcommittee in formal mark-up sessions being significantly less controversial than the original administration bill, although there were still many points in contention.

The Issues—Retroactivity and the Double Ratchet

In meeting with congressmen and staff, Irv Wolkstein and other AHA representatives had hit hard on the issue of applying a revenue limit to the 1976 base year, and the inequity of applying the adjustments necessary to bring the revenue limit forward to the control period on an additive basis. This would mean that the rate actually allowed the hospital in the intervening period would be less than the maximum 15 percent stated in the administration bill. Moreover, the limit was being applied after the fact, and AHA pointed out that any hospital whose rate of inflation exceeded the rate allowed in the intervening period would necessarily be held to a rate of increase significantly less than 9 percent of the first year of controls.

In an effort to ameliorate the effect of this provision, Rogers proposed that during the intervening period the hospital be allowed its actual rate of inflation (as in the administration's bill) but that the limits be set at a minimum of 9 percent inflation and a maximum of 20 percent, instead of 6 and 15 percent, respectively. HEW pointed out that the Rogers proposal would reduce the savings produced by the program by 25 percent, and Rogers partially backed away from the proposal, leaving the upper limit at 15 percent with a lower limit of 9.

In a further attempt to soften the effect of the program and thereby make it more defensible, Rogers proposed that the double ratchet effect be removed. The administration had proposed to institute a declining revenue limit applied on an additive basis to base year revenue. Again, AHA pushed hard on the inequity of the administration's approach and even supplied the subcommittee members with a chart which demonstrated that the actual allowable rate of inflation under the administration's proposal would be less than the 6 percent GNP deflator by the third year of the program. The Rogers proposal deleted this effect by providing that the revenue increase limit would be equal to 1.5 times the GNP deflator, and would be applied to the previous year's revenue. This change in the limit and the use of compounding met immediate approval from the subcommittee members. After all, it was a lot easier to say, as Rogers did, that the proposal would allow hospitals a rate 50 percent higher than the rate experienced by the rest of the economy than it was to defend a declining limit which was less than the secretary of HEW had said it was. HEW argued again that subcommittee approval of the Rogers proposal would mean substantially lower savings, but the important point was that, with the change, the subcommittee had removed AHA's major argument against the bill. In fact, the subcommittee liked the idea of compounding the allowable rate of increase so much that it later returned to the question of the rate allowed in the intervening period and decided to compound that too, although the maximum total increase in the two-year period between the base year and the first control year could be no higher than 30 percent.

Inflation in the Hospital "Market Basket"

Although the subcommittee decided to allow a more generous rate of inflation than the administration had proposed, there was still a great deal of uncertainty expressed, especially by Congressman Carter, on the effects of the limit on needed hospital services. This concern was directly connected to AHA's claim that its cost index "proved" that inflation in hospitals was primarily a function of higher input prices. In consideration of this concern, the subcommittee included a provision originally contained in Carter's bill which directed the secretary of HEW to develop and provide to the Congress by March 31, 1979, an index that reflects the prices of the components of hospital costs. Carter had wanted to mandate the use of the index at that point but HEW argued against it, noting the difficulty in producing the index and, therefore, the subcommittee compromised by requiring the secretary to provide recommendations concerning whether such an index should replace the revenue limit based upon the GNP deflator.

Comment. These first two issues are the best examples of the general tone of the changes to the administration's bill accepted by the subcommittee. First, a great deal of uncertainty about the impact of the administration's proposal, and a dearth of data with which to discern that impact, led the subcommittee to loosen the provisions of the bill in several instances. Second, the uncertainty and lack of data led the subcommittee to include in its bill a series of instructions to the secretary concerning the development of answers to many questions raised by the subcommittee's deliberations. For example, where the original administration's bill had directed the secretary to develop a report on permanent reforms, the subcommittee bill directed the secretary to report on the price index, progress in the development of uniform accounting and reporting systems, establishment of a system of classification of hospitals, a permanent method for the reduction of capacity, the appropriate roles of HSAs and PSROs in cost containment activities, and the determination of rates of reimbursement based upon case mix. The administration had proposed that use of the wage pass-through after September 1, 1979 be at the discretion of the secretary; the subcommittee bill directed the secretary to report on the experience with the pass-through, its effect on wages, and the secretary's recommendations on its use, with the Congress having veto power over the secretary's decision. Concerning the Title II capital expenditure limitations, the subcommittee bill required a report from the secretary on whether the $2.5 billion limit was adequate; a report from the secretary was also required concerning the effects of the limit upon its application.

In effect these actions were the methods used by the subcommittee to reconcile extensive concern about the effects of unrestrained inflation in hospital care, and the equally important concern about the impact of revenue and capital limits on the delivery of needed health care services. Although some of that concern over impact was lessened by softening some of the provisions of the bill, the intent of the subcommittee was to institute the controls on a trial basis, require HEW to study their impact, and then modify the program at a later date if the legislation proved to be wrong. Many of the provisions modified or added to the bill reflect this essential point.

Admission Load Adjustment

The administration's bill had proposed that the total revenue limit be adjusted upward for each admission above 102 percent of base year admissions by an amount equal to 50 percent of the average reimbursement (or charge) per admission. Although the adjustment was designed to reduce incentives toward increased volume by assuring that only variable costs associated with an additional admission were recognized, the administration's proposal in this regard was not well received by the subcommittee. The first problem faced by HEW was to explain the notion of fixed and variable costs to the congressmen. Next, HEW had to explain why, at a certain volume level, the hospital's fixed costs were essentially covered, which meant that if the reimbursement limit for admissions near that level were pegged at full average reimbursement, the hospital would make a profit on increased volume; this could be an incentive to inappropriately increase volume. Unfortunately for HEW, it was clear that its arguments were not getting through; Congressmen Satterfield and Carter repeatedly asked why HEW wanted some patients to pay the full rate, while others paid only half. HEW responded by pointing out that the provision did not mean that at all; it meant that if volume projections showed that admissions would rise above the base year level, the hospital would have to reduce the revenue it received for each patient so that it would stay within the total allowable revenue limit as adjusted by the admission load formula.

Congressman Andrew Maguire (D.-N.J.) raised a more sophisticated point. Maguire and his staff had researched the question of the relationship of fixed to variable costs, and concluded that the 50 percent reduction was not indicated by their research. HEW argued otherwise but, again, the uncertainty was there and HEW did not provide data sufficient to erase it. The result was another study on the extent to which the allowance reflects statistical indicators of costs related to the efficient production of hospital services.

Exemptions for State Cost Containment Programs

As a result of Carter's strong support for state cost containment programs, as well as the desire of Rogers to accommodate Carter's point of view, the subcommittee bill contains the strongest expression of support for state programs included in any of the bills considered by any of the concerned subcommittees. Partial recognition for the strength of the state exemption section lies with the knowledge that one of Rogers's staff persons had worked as a consultant to the Maryland rate review commission and was very sympathetic to Carter's points on state programs, especially in regard to the need for linkage of revenue limitation programs to health planning and to utilization review and quality assurance.

In fact, the major problem faced by majority and minority staff was not in reaching a compromise between Carter and Rogers, but in designing a mutually acceptable program about which HEW would not be totally negative. For example, Rogers had proposed to delete the administration's requirement that state programs be in operation for one year, and had also proposed that the standard under which state performance would be judged be 120 percent of the promulgated limit under the federal program. Both proposals were in line with the minority's wishes, but Carter also wanted to remove the requirement that the states have a plan approved by the secretary for recovery of any excess revenue. Carter's staff argued that the requirement gave the secretary too much power over the operation of state programs, but HEW argued that it was the only way it could insure that the state would actually run an effective program. Moreover, HEW indicated that if it had to it would accept the deletion of the one-year operational requirement and the use of the higher revenue standard, but it insisted that each state program have a plan to recover excess revenue. The need for compromise dictated that this last requirement stay in the bill.

When it came to the question of linkage, there was no disagreement whatsoever; the language from Carter's proposal was inserted into the bill essentially unchanged, and was made a requirement for all state programs. As in the Kennedy subcommittee, Carter's proposals on the administrative structure of new state cost containment programs were added as a new section, and federal funding for state programs was provided for these states which met the requirements. HEW asked that authority for the secretary to change the requirements at a future point be included but, again, the minority argued that such authority conveyed too much power to HEW. Compromise was reached by allowing the secretary to modify or waive the requirements. but not to add to them.

An amendment was offered by Representative Henry A. Waxman (D.-Calif.) which required states to exempt HMO hospitals, as did the federal program. Some discussion ensued as to whether or not this requirement constituted a more stringent standard for states since HMO hospitals would presumably be at the lower end of the cost increase spectrum and exclusion of them from a state program would, therefore, increase the statewide average. Again, the data needed to answer this question definitively were not available; moreover, California-based Kaiser-Permanente, the country's largest HMO, maintains a full-time lobbyist in Washington and Kaiser had worked diligently lining up support for the Waxman amendment.

The major thing which the subcommittee did not include in the state exemption section was a provision similar to the Kennedy subcommittee's provision requiring the use of a wage pass-through in state programs. In preliminary discussions, Waxman had indicated that he would offer such an amendment and Carter and his staff had geared up to argue against it. But, perhaps because of the more business-oriented stance of the Commerce Committee, or because of the influence of the majority staff person who had worked with the Maryland program, Waxman never offered the amendment.

Other Title I Issues

The subcommittee extensively revised the language of many other sections in Title I and added several other new proposals designed to deal with its concerns about the health care delivery system. Carter's proposal to encourage the consolidation of hospital services was included, as was Rogers' proposal to provide some financial incentives for "good" behavior. Significant additions were made to the exceptions process. The test of financial need was changed from requiring the hospital to be in the lowest 25 percent of all hospitals in regard to its current ratio of assets and liabilities to the flat requirement that the current ratio of assets to liabilities be less than two. A hospital with increased admissions of higher than 15 percent or a substantial change in capacity because of being in a growth area, or a hospital with a substantial change in capacity due to the closing of another hospital in the area, would not be required to meet the current ratio test. In a significant change from the administration's bill, the subcommittee decided that hospitals which were sole community providers, and which were found to be needed by the HSA, would be eligible for an exception solely on the basis of financial need if their current asset to liability ratio fell below two to one, i.e., two dollars of current assets to one dollar of current liability.

The greatest amount of discussion concerning the exceptions process focused on the definition of "asset" for purposes of the current ratio. The issue originally was raised by the Hospital Financial Development Association (HFDA), which pointed out that inclusion of unrestricted donations in the definition of the current ratio would force hospitals in need of an exception to expend all of the unrestricted donations, as well as any proceeds from previously donated property. The administration's bill excluded restricted gifts. HFDA maintained that including unrestricted donations in the definition of the current ratio would result in a significant reduction in voluntary donations to hospitals. Its most compelling argument was that if donations were to dry up, the funding would have to come from somewhere, and that most likely would be the federal government.

It should be pointed out that $4 billion were donated to hospitals in 1976, according to HFDA. Carter proposed an amendment excluding all donations from the current ratio test, and the subcommittee agreed. One thing was clear, a well-organized lobbying campaign had insured passage of the amendment before it was offered.

With little controversy or discussion, the subcommittee also excluded from the transitional revenue limitation program all hospitals with less than 4,000 admissions which also were sole providers to a community. In addition, strict financial disclosure requirements were imposed on hospitals and common audits were mandated for the Medicare and Medicaid programs.

Another issue which lead to some controversy was the subcommittee's decision to allow small rural hospitals to use beds on a "swing" basis as long-term care beds or acute care beds, as needed. The American Health Care Association, the professional association of long-term care providers, argued that "it is questionable whether conversion of hospital beds is a less expensive way to provide long-term care services than construction of a free-standing facility."[6] Since the subcommittee limited reimbursement for these long-term swing beds to the average found in free-standing long-term facilities, this was not thought to be a problem.

The only other section of Title I about which there was some controversy was Rogers' and HEW's proposal to outlaw totally percentage arrangements used to pay certain physicians, normally radiologists and pathologists. The College of American Pathologists retorted that it was aware of the abuses that had occurred as a result of these arrangements, but that no hearings had ever been held and, therefore, there had been no exploration of alternative methods of payment. Carter pointed out that in his rural district, percentage arrangements were the only way to get certain services such as pathology, and he wanted to know what HEW proposed to do if those arrangements were outlawed. As expected, a compromise was reached in which compensation paid to a physician could not be based upon a rental, lease, or finder's fee, but could be based upon a percentage of revenue received for a radiology or pathology department, for example, as long as the total compensation did not exceed the amount the physician could "reasonably" have expected to receive if the physician were paid a salary plus "reasonable expenses."

Title II—Issues Concerning the Capital Expenditure Limitations

The Title II provisions agreed to by the subcommittee were essentially the provisions originally proposed by H.R. 8121, described in Chapter 7. The $2.5 billion limit, the supply standard, and the occupancy standard were included in the subcommittee's bill as well as the changes proposed to make consistent the certificate of need provisions of Section 1122 of the Social Security Act and the National Health Planning Act. Special consideration of national health resource centers also was included as proposed by both the Rogers and Carter bills.

With little controversy, changes were made in the conditions under which health systems agencies (HSAs) and state level health planning agencies could approve the construction of hospital beds in areas with too many beds or too low an occupancy. The administration had proposed that approval of new bed construction could only occur on the basis of one new bed for every two that were permanently closed. The subcommittee added to that condition by allowing the construction of new beds for HMO hospitals if the state agency found that the existing supply of hospital beds would not appropriately meet the needs of an HMO, and by allowing new construction in a "subpart" of the health service area if that subpart was in compliance with the standards and the new construction was needed for compliance with various codes and accreditation standards.

Discussion on Title II took place on the question of whether or not $2.5 billion was adequate. As was noted in Chapter 5, the HEW people never provided Congress with a reasonable defense of the $2.5 billion limit and, therefore, the strong suspicion left was that they had pulled the figure out of their hat. The subcommittee agreed to Rogers' proposal to raise the limit each year by the existing annual inflation rate in the costs of construction; however, the basic response to the problem was to order another study by HEW on the effects of the limit.

At this time, Title II had yet to engender the amount of controversy associated with Title I. Except for the large manufacturers of medical equipment, there were no lobbyists hammering away at the "inequity" of the proposed capital expenditure limitations as AHA and FAH had done in regard to the proposed revenue limitations.

The one issue which caused what can be termed a controversy within the subcommittee was the question of extending the certificate of need program to the purchase of medical equipment for physician's offices and clinics. Rogers's inclusion of such an extension in H.R. 8121, and in the subcommittee's working drafts, caused the AMA to be concerned and it increased its active lobbying efforts against the bill. As the subcommittee approached the point at which it would take up the medical equipment question, letters and telegrams from doctors and medical societies began to pour in. One day before discussion on the issue was to occur, the AMA's chief Washington lobbyist, John Zapp, made the rounds of the congressional offices. The result was a discussion between Rogers and Carter early the next morning which ended with Carter's turning to his staff and requesting the proper language for deleting the medical equipment provisions from the bill.

The vote on the amendment was rather comical as Carter offered it as a substitute to an amendment proposed by Waxman. Waxman, at the behest of the American Clinical Laboratory Association, was in the process of offering an amendment to exclude clinical laboratory equipment from the proposed new certificate of need authority. Carter essentially went Waxman one better by offering a substitute amendment to exclude *all* noninstitutional equipment. The vote was taken on Carter's substitute first and, when the chairman asked for the yeas and nays, only Carter voted in favor of it. Carter quickly noted that there would not be a quorum if he left the meeting room, and prepared to leave, thereby making the vote nonbinding. In the confusion, Rogers asked for the negative votes and it turned out that there were none and Carter's substitute carried. When Carter realized that he had won, he returned and the vote was taken on the Waxman amendment as modified by the Carter amendment. The end result was that no one, except Carter and Rogers, realized quite what had happened and heads were turning all around the room in an attempt to ascertain whether or not the subcommittee had in fact just deleted the medical equipment provisions of the bill. Of course, what both the spectators and the staff did not know was that Carter had told Rogers that he just could not support the bill if the medical equipment provisions were left in it, and Rogers had agreed in advance to recede on the issue. Rogers did not give up on the extension of certificate of need; it appeared again in his proposed amendments to the health planning bill which was considered by the subcommittee in March 1978.

Title III—Support for Closure or Conversion of Excess Capacity

By the time the subcommittee reached consideration of Title III attendance had dropped off. It was clear that the subcommittee members had heard all they wanted on the subject of cost containment, at least for a while. Consideration of Title III was relatively brief, and it was agreed to with few changes in the form originally proposed by Rogers in H.R. 8121. The only outstanding question was whether the 5 percent reduction in federal reimbursement originally proposed by Rogers was too severe for hospitals which the HSA had identified as maintaining excess capacity or for those identified as not needed. Since discussion on the penalty occurred at the end of almost a solid month of discussion on cost containment, the penalty issue was never fully explored. Instead, it seemed that members of the subcommittee relied upon the judgment of the chairman on this issue, and so the "voluntary" program to reduce excess capacity continued to mandate a penalty for noncompliance.

Celebration

As Chairman Rogers turned to the members of the subcommittee present and asked who would cosponsor a "clean" version of the bill for distribution to other members of the House, it seemed as if one of the major hurdles in getting a cost containment bill through the Congress had just been passed. With all of the members present agreeing to cosponsor the bill (introduced as H.R. 9717), and with HEW staff coming forward to congratulate the members and staff on their efforts, the problems of getting a bill through Ways and Means in the House and through Finance in the Senate seemed small indeed. However, there were many other congressmen, both on the other committees responsible for the bill and on the Health and the Environment Subcommittee's own full Committee on Interstate and Foreign Commerce, who had not partici-pated in the debate up to this time and who did not agree at all with the sentiments expressed by Chairman Rogers in a letter to colleagues on October 21, 1977: "I believe that the substitute amendment reported by the Subcommittee contains a number of significant improvements over the original legislation proposed by the Administration. Without sacri-ficing the realization of significant savings, the proposal has been made more workable and considerably more palatable to the hospitals which will be affected."[7] Dr. Carter also was hopeful that the changes proposed by the subcommittee would be met with approval by the Amer-ican Hospital Association, and directed his staff to talk with AHA staff about their reactions to H.R. 9717. Carter's staff spoke to Michael Hash of AHA and were told that the association was very appreciative of Carter's efforts, particularly in regard to the state exemptions and for reducing the inequities in the original revenue increase limit formula. Nevertheless, Hash stated that AHA would continue to oppose the bill publicly to the best of its ability.[8]

As the focus of cost containment efforts shifted away from the Sub-committee on Health and the Environment, AHA's opposition to the subcommittee's actions was not to be the real problem. After all, it probably was not reasonable to expect a hospital association to support any hospital cost containment bill, no matter what softening of provi-sions had occurred. As the next chapter describes, the significant

problem for proponents of the basic thrust of the administration's bill
was that Rostenkowski decided that the bill could not pass the Ways and
Means Committee unless it was radically altered. The bombshell dropped
by Rostenkowski when he proposed his alternative was to change totally
the shape of the congressional response to hospital cost containment.

9 | The Voluntary Effort

As the end of the first session of the 95th Congress drew near, it became obvious that no further action would be taken on cost containment before Congress returned in January. Both the Committee on Ways and Means, and the Committee on Interstate and Foreign Commerce were deeply involved in the president's energy bill. Senator Talmadge had not budged from his earlier position, and Rostenkowski had suspended "indefinitely" mark-up sessions in his subcommittee. The president seemed to acknowledge this reality when, at the signing of the Medicare-Medicaid Anti-Fraud and Abuse Bill on October 25, 1977, he expressed hope that "we can all return next year" for the signing of cost containment legislation.[1]

Nonetheless, the administration did not seem to be particularly unhappy with the progress achieved by that time. The two health subcommittees which handle virtually all federal health legislation, other than Medicare in the House and other than Medicare and Medicaid in the Senate, had approved legislation substantially similar to the administration's original proposal. The prevailing wisdom was that Rostenkowski would move forward as soon as consideration of the energy and Social Security legislation was complete, and that the combination of forces would then move Talmadge to act. A score card was needed at this point to keep straight all of the varying alternatives, but it seemed that the long process of deliberation and negotiation inherent in moving the bill through the full committees, on to the respective floors, and into a conference between House and Senate would provide an opportunity to rectify the different proposals. In fact, informal staff-level meetings were already occurring at this point in an effort to sketch out the broad outlines of the needed compromises.

There were some signs, however, that the situation was not progressing as the administration had hoped. Congressmen James T. Broyhill (R.-N.C.) and Edward R. Madigan (R.-Ill.) of the Commerce Health Subcommittee had let it be known that they were going to offer an amendment in the full Commerce Committee to strike Title I (the revenue limitations), and AHA was trying to obtain support for their move. Regardless, this move was not unexpected from two Republican congressmen, and it still looked as if the administration would prevail. A more important signal of things to come was included in a statement presented to the House by Congressman Daniel Rostenkowski on November 2, 1977, in which he noted the difficulties his subcommittee had been experiencing with the administration's proposal. His statement hinted at future developments:

> Since mid-May my own Ways and Means Subcommittee on Health has given intense, if periodic, consideration to the issue. Unfortunately, the need to devote attention to other high-priority legislation, as well as some dissatisfaction among members with aspects of the Administration's hospital cost containment bill, have precluded my Subcommittee from completing its consideration of possible solutions to the health cost escalation problem. . . .
>
> I believe that the period between now and the reconvening of Congress in January can be well spent by both the Administration and the hospital industry in determining the best direction to take in achieving a means of containing hospital costs. For the Administration it is a time to reassess its proposal, and to modify it where appropriate and to strengthen support for it both in the public and in the Congress. And because Congress has not passed legislation on the subject this year, the hospitals in this country have been given a brief grace period. With the knowledge that we will not resume consideration of the issue until early next year, *hospitals have the opportunity to demonstrate that they can finally take the initiative and effectively and significantly restrain cost increases on a voluntary basis.*
>
> Furthermore, *as I have stated to representatives of the American Hospital Association, the Federation of American Hospitals, and the American Medical Association,* I hope the entire private sector will accept this *challenge* to develop a meaningful program of cost containment. . .
>
> In stating that the private sector should take the initiative, however, I do not seek nor am I in a position to accept unnecessary delay in consideration of the Administration's proposal next year. The industry has had a cost problem for years but has not been able to deal effectively with it without Government involvement. *If the industry is as confident as their representatives have indicated to me that they can solve the hospital cost problem on a voluntary basis, they should be in a position to develop and to begin to implement a responsible alternative before congressional debate on this issue resumes in February.*[2] [Emphasis added.]

Answering the Rostenkowski "Challenge"

The AHA, FAH and AMA moved quickly to answer the Rostenkowski challenge. Within three weeks a National Steering Committee on Voluntary Cost Containment had been established, and on November 23, 1977 AHA sent mailgrams to its members calling for "an immediate reassessment by each institution of planned budget and charge adjustments...to see if anything further can be done in the short term to reduce these increases."[3] By December 20, 1977, the steering committee had met and agreed upon general outlines of the voluntary program and a national goal of a 2 percent reduction in the rate of increase of hospital costs in both 1978 and 1979.

In consideration of the long-term nature of inflation in hospital costs, and the paucity of previous serious efforts by the private sector to address the problem, it was naturally surprising that these three organizations could move so fast in answering Rostenkowski's challenge. As might be expected, the entire effort had been orchestrated in advance with the original impetus for the voluntary plan coming from the Federation of American Hospitals.[4] Therefore, when Rostenkowski saw that it would be difficult, if not impossible, to get the administration's bill through his subcommittee, as demonstrated by the close votes taken by the subcommittee in its July deliberations, the lobbyists were ready with an alternative. His "challenge" was actually an acceptance by Rostenkowski of that alternative, although at this point the three organizations still had to come through with the actual machinery to implement a voluntary effort.

The Voluntary Effort

By early January, an office for the voluntary hospital cost containment program was established at AHA's offices in Chicago, and a futuristic "Voluntary Effort" logo had been designed and stationery printed. Letters were sent to every hospital board chairman, executive officer, and medical staff chief. On January 16, 1978, the program was officially announced to the public, and within two weeks about 40 states had formed state voluntary cost containment committees. There could be no questions now that the three organizations had been ready and willing to implement the proposed alternative, and that they had been highly successful in doing so.

The program proposed by the Voluntary Effort was fairly simple. First, it established the goal of a 2 percent annual reduction in hospital cost increases in 1978 and 1979. Second, it proposed that there be no net increase in hospital beds in 1978. Third, hospitals were to reduce the rate of total capital expenditures to 80 percent of the price-adjusted 1975 through 1977 average of hospital capital investment. Implementation of the program would be accomplished primarily at the state level through the voluntary cost containment committees. Although it was proposed that states be given flexibility in implementing the objectives, the National Steering Committee suggested that states either: (1) screen for those hospitals within the state which were in the top 15 percent (or some comparable percentage) of growth in revenue or cost per admission; or (2) review hospitals that had a rate of increase of more than 10 percent (or some comparable percentage) in revenues or cost per admission in 1978 as compared to fiscal 1977; and (3) for all states, screen any hospital that had a rate of increase in its total budgeted revenues or expenditures that was not at least 2 percent below the rate of increase compared to the last fiscal year. The national committee was somewhat less explicit about how the state committees were to achieve the capital expenditure goal. The state committees were asked only to establish a state goal for hospital capital expenditures "in light of the national goal but reflecting the special needs of their area."[5] The national committee then would review each state capital expenditure goal.

The Rostenkowski Response

On February 1, 1978, Rostenkowski responded to the efforts of AHA, AMA, and FAH in implementing the structure of the Voluntary Effort in a speech before the House of Delegates of the American Hospital Association. Referring to his November 2 statement, and the challenge contained therein, Rostenkowski said: "I am heartened to see that the challenge has been accepted. I am pleased by the seriousness of purpose and the delineation of goals of the so-called 'Voluntary Effort.' You have acted with all deliberate speed to establish principles and propose a national mechanism which has the potential of translating these principles into tangible results. Even your harshest critics must be impressed with these early efforts.... In a sense the impact of President Carter's nine percent cap solution could be paralleled to the impact of the old Selective Service System. Nothing stimulates volunteers more quickly than the fear of a draft."[6]

Nonetheless, Rostenkowski was not totally convinced that the new voluntary program would achieve the goals which it had set forth for itself: "To accommodate the possibility, however remote, that the Voluntary Effort falls short of its goals, I shall ask my Subcommittee to develop a legislative proposal which would include only standby hospital cost controls. These would be modeled on the President's original proposal but they would be implemented only if the rate of increase in hospital costs did not decline by two percent in 1978 or by an additional two percent in 1979."[7]

Thus, in what has been termed a "masterful" stroke,[8] Rostenkowski changed all the rules of the congressional consideration of hospital cost containment. As noted by the *National Journal,* the rationale for Rostenkowski's move was quite sound: "[Rostenkowski] and his staff argue that the Administration's original measure was destined for oblivion and its only hope was to place the onus for cost reductions on hospitals and doctors. Now that these interests have developed a voluntary containment plan, they cannot complain about standby federal controls if their scheme fails."[9]

However, neither the administration nor the hospitals warmly embraced Rostenkowski's move, with the congressman noting on February 8 that "such mutual reluctance is encouraging for it might well serve as the basis for a viable compromise."[10] In fact, the administration did not particularly oppose the new proposal, most likely because it accepted the judgment of Rostenkowski that his move was necessary if the bill was to pass. Rostenkowski met with the president late in February, and President Carter reportedly stated that he would accept a cost containment bill in any form.[11] In any case, given the time lag before a mandatory program similar to the one approved by the Commerce Health Subcommittee could start, the cost savings under Rostenkowski's plan and the mandatory program were not all that far apart. It was evidently more important to the administration to get Congress on record in favor of some kind of restraints on hospital cost increases than it was to quibble over the form of the program.

Significant opposition to the Rostenkowski proposal came from the hospital lobbyists, AMA, and labor. The hospital lobbyists and AMA opposed the proposal because it was more likely to pass, and because they felt that standby controls would undercut the voluntary program. AHA Vice President Paul Earle claimed that standby controls would create an incentive for hospital administrators to increase their costs during the base year against which mandatory controls would be applied. Earle predicted that such an economic incentive would cause administrators to ignore the voluntary controls so that they would not be in a tight financial position when and if controls were imposed.[12]

Labor opposed the Rostenkowski proposal because it felt that the most likely method hospital administrators would find to meet the goals of the Voluntary Effort was to reduce wages.[13] The administration's bill had provided some protection for labor, and the Kennedy subcommittee had gone even further, but there was no such protection included in the Voluntary Effort's statements about the structure of its program. In the face of these efforts by labor and by the provider lobbies, Rostenkowski scheduled mark-up activities for his subcommittee late in February and the debate in Congress over cost containment heated up once again.

Subcommittee Mark-Up—Ways and Means

Although Rostenkowski had proposed his compromise with an explicit purpose of reducing the opposition to cost containment in his subcommittee, the discussions in the subcommittee and the closeness of the final vote indicated little achievement in that regard. White House health aide Joseph Onek indicated that the administration had pulled out all the stops in lobbying for the bill, but Rostenkowski was only able to muster 7 affirmative votes out of 13 when the final vote to report the bill was taken.[14] Moreover, Republican members of the subcommittee, joined by Democrats Otis G. Pike (New York) and Omar Burleson (Texas), offered a series of amendments designed to soften significantly the provisions of the standby mandatory program, much as they had attempted to do in the subcommittee's earlier sessions held in July 1977.

Of these minority proposals, the subcommittee agreed to amendments offered by Willis D. Gradison, Jr., (R.-Ohio) to provide for pass-throughs for energy and malpractice insurance costs, although the subcommittee did not accept Gradison's proposed pass-throughs for food, social security, unemployment compensation payments, pensions, depreciation, and interest costs. The subcommittee also did not accept an amendment offered by James G. Martin (R.-N.C.) to require joint approval by both houses of Congress before a mandatory program could go into effect, or a later Martin amendment providing each house of Congress with a right to veto the mandatory program. Also voted down was a Gradison proposal that states meeting the voluntary goals be exempt from any mandatory program, a proposal which was to surface later in the Commerce Committee and the Senate.

Despite the efforts of Gradison and others, the subcommittee finally reported a bill to the full Ways and Means Committee on February 28, 1978 on a 7 to 6 vote. Except for the pass-throughs for energy and malpractice, the standby part of the program was very similar to the mandatory program agreed to by the Commerce Health Subcommittee. The subcommittee agreed to an amendment offered by John J. Duncan (R.-Tenn.) which broadened the options for state programs. It incorporated the revised revenue limit and the hospital costs index included in the Commerce bill, as well as the exclusion for small hospitals which were sole community providers. Also, despite the best efforts of labor, the subcommittee chose not to make the wage pass-through mandatory nor to require states to include it in their programs. The only significant differences between the bill reported by the Ways and Means subcommittee and the Commerce subcommittee were the standby nature of the federal controls, the inclusion of federal hospitals in the revenue limitation program (a provision Commerce had been unable to include), and Rostenkowski's exclusion of all of the capital expenditure controls and excess capacity reduction proposals embodied in Titles II and III of the Commerce bill, on the grounds that those provisions were not within Ways and Means' jurisdiction.

Conclusion

With the action of the Ways and Means subcommittee in approving the Rostenkowski compromise in late February, the prospects for approval of some form of cost containment were looking up, although approval was by no means assured. It was not clear how Rogers would proceed in the full Committee on Interstate and Foreign Commerce, but it was hard to see how Rogers could avoid including the standby aspects of the Rostenkowski proposal in the bill reported by the full Commerce Committee. After all, it is very difficult to be a proponent of mandatory controls when an equally important member of the congressional health establishment has already agreed to a voluntary program with only standby controls. A significant question was whether or not the business-oriented Commerce Committee would accept AHA's strenuous arguments about the inequity of the program and the improper incentives associated with the standby controls.

Various reports credited Rostenkowski with having the votes to get the bill through the full Ways and Means Committee, although again approval was not certain.[15] The small size of the margin Rostenkowski was able to obtain in his subcommittee indicated that passage by the full committee would be a difficult process.

As Congress returned from its spring recess ending April 3, 1978, both subcommittee chairmen had prepared an attempt to obtain approval from their respective full committees, but the question still outstanding was what Senator Talmadge would do with cost containment. By refusing to act on the administration's proposal, Talmadge was holding all of the cards and was in a position to demand compromises from the administration. Talmadge had scheduled mark-up sessions on his bill, and staffs from HEW, Kennedy's subcommittee, and the House were negotiating with Talmadge's staff in an attempt to find a compromise.

The larger question facing the committees was whether to accept the Voluntary Effort. It was necessary to assess whether or not it was workable; its success would preclude the necessity of pushing ahead through the political morass in which Congress was embroiled.

First, the Voluntary Effort could be construed as an attempt to perpetuate the status quo, rather than a voluntary attempt to implement the intent of the administration's proposal. The administration had proposed that the rate of increase in hospital costs be brought close to or below the rate of increase in prices in the general economy. The primary basis for the proposal was that the opportunity costs of hospital care (the costs of those other improvements in health care lost because so much revenue is consumed by hospitals) are very high, especially in consideration of evidence which suggests that health status could be improved more reliably if health care resources were committed to primary care, environmental safeguards, childhood immunizations, and other noninstitutional activities. In contrast, the Voluntary Effort organizations stated that the basis for the proposed two-year, 2 percent per year reduction was to reduce the 15.6 percent rate of inflation in hospital costs closer to the present 10.8 percent rate of growth in GNP. Moreover, the Voluntary Effort proposed to hold the line after the 4 percent reduction was achieved. On top of a static 11.6 percent rate, .8 percent above the present growth in total GNP, the Voluntary Effort further proposed to adjust the goal for unforeseen changes (e.g., energy) in input costs.

The Voluntary Effort did not propose to institute any actions to remove the present maldistribution of capacity by removing expensive and unneeded excess capacity or by encouraging the construction of capacity in underserved areas. The Voluntary Effort proposed a freeze on new beds and a 20 percent reduction in capital expenditures, although it is not clear whether the 20 percent referred to nonbed expenditures or to total expenditures. Current bed construction accounts for 23 percent of total capital expenditures, so the goal actually may envision an increase in nonbed items.

Another reason for concern about the Voluntary Effort is that any nongovernmental scheme which establishes a target rate may be found to be in violation of the antitrust laws. The Voluntary Effort had requested a "business review" or antitrust clearance from the Justice Department but the Anti-Trust Division of the Department declined to grant the request. The June 12th statement from the Justice Department noted that "our present understanding of this complex [health care] industry precludes a definitive analysis," and "accordingly, we must decline your request for a statement of our enforcement intentions."[16] Essentially, this response meant that Justice was reserving the right to proceed with an antitrust action at any future time.

It was also possible that the Justice Department's decision may not have been based totally on technical considerations. On May 10, 1978, HEW General Counsel Peter Libassi wrote the Justice Department to request that a decision on an antitrust exemption for the Voluntary Effort be deferred. Libassi stated in his letter that state Voluntary Effort Committee activities might have significant adverse effects on health services through discrimination against smaller hospitals, or HMOs or through inappropriate controls on hospital workers' wages.[17] The Voluntary Effort denied Libassi's contentions and claimed that his letter was "a political maneuver consistent with the Administration's inconsistency in dealing with health policy."[18] Libassi's concerns, however, were further substantitated by Federal Trade Commission Chairman Michael Pertschuk in a letter to Representative John Moss (D.-Calif.) which expressed Pertschuk's doubts that a provider-dominated program could act in the public interest.[19]

Nevertheless, even though these concerns about the long-term implications of the Voluntary Effort may persist, the program did appear to be enjoying some success during its first several months of operation. By May 1978, the rate of increase in hospital expenditures had dropped to an annual rate of 12.6 percent according to AHA's National Panel Survey.[20] Even more importantly, the overall Consumer Price Index had been rising faster than the medical care and hospital care segments of the CPI from March through June of 1978.[21] The June CPI figures showed all prices increasing by .9 percent with the prices for medical care and for hospitals rising .5 percent and .2 percent respectively. Thus, these data gave the providers solid evidence with which to refute the arguments of the administration and the supporters of a mandatory cost containment program that a voluntary program would not work. The success of the providers in structuring what appeared to be a sound alternative to the mandatory plan was to have far-reaching implications as consideration of cost containment legislation proceeded in Congress.

10 | The Failure of the Cost Containment Effort

House Action

The Rogers Substitute

On May 17, 1978, Chairman Rogers of the Subcommittee on Health and the Environment sent each member of the full Interstate and Foreign Commerce Committee a "Dear Colleague" letter describing the substitute cost containment bill which Rogers intended to introduce at the Committee's cost containment mark-up scheduled for the following week. The letter represented an attempt to compromise between both the expressed concerns of the provider lobbies and the proposals of Rostenkowski and Talmadge, and was the culmination of several weeks of negotiation and discussion. Apparently, Rogers and Rostenkowski had met in Puerto Rico at a medical device industry convention in February, and decided to seek a compromise in an effort to gain support for the bill.[1]

Rogers's letter pointed out that Rostenkowski's "proposal has much to recommend it, and my amendment would incorporate the substance of the Rostenkowski approach."[2] In fact, the only major differences between Rogers's proposed substitute and the Ways and Means Subcommittee reported bill were a statement of principles for hospital reimbursement reform and changes in Titles II and III which Rostenkowski had not addressed. The statement on principles for long-term reform arose from "discussions between the Administration, Senator Talmadge, and [Rogers]," and would include "changes in Medicare and Medicaid to classify hospitals based upon the nature and intensity of the services they provide and to pay them based upon their comparative performance, with an incentive system for those who perform well; opportunities for effective state systems to operate in place of a Federal control program; and the development of a method for limiting increases in hospital revenues which reflects prevailing wage levels, the price of items which constitute components of hospital costs, and the marginal costs to hospitals resulting from changes in admissions."[3] Rogers noted that much of this reform could not be accomplished immediately, so the substitute proposed to establish an independent commission which would assist the secretary in developing the methodology and data to make these reforms feasible. The substitute further provided the secretary with authority to institute the reforms as soon as the methodologies were available, subject to a congressional veto.

Rogers also proposed to make significant changes in Titles II and III of the bill, the capital expenditures limitation and the program to reduce excess hospital capacity. First, the capital limit was to be raised from $2.5 billion to $3 billion; second, the hospital bed supply (four beds per 1000 population) and the occupancy (minimum of 80 percent) standards were to be deleted; and third, the penalty for failure to close an unneeded facility through Title III was to be deleted. It should be noted that in proposing his substitute Rogers was attempting to respond directly to the providers and to Talmadge. The statement of principles essentially embodied the methodology contained in Talmadge's bill (S. 1470) and, in a sense, responded to providers' criticism of the bill. As stated by Rogers, "I believe that this approach responds to the concerns of those who say that the transitional program does not take account of differences in hospitals, the costs of the goods they purchase, and different wage situations."[4] Through increasing the capital expenditures limit and deleting the rigid standards and penalties, it was clear that Rogers was weakening the original bill but was addressing the controversy concerning rigid supply standards which rose during the subcommittee's discussion of the Health Planning Amendments of 1978.[5]

Unfortunately, Rogers's efforts to lessen provider criticism and to achieve a consensus with Senator Talmadge were not immediately apparent. The senator's Subcommittee on Health of the Finance Committee scheduled mark-up on S. 1470 for June 20 while the Commerce Committee was still deliberating the Rogers substitute. The three major provider lobbies (the American Hospital Association, the American Medical Association, and the Federation of American Hospitals) also responded negatively to the proposed substitute through letters sent to Rogers and to the other committee members.[6] The letters noted that instituting stand-by controls would interfere with the Voluntary Effort by permitting revenues, in anticipation of mandatory controls, to be raised to the maximum levels allowed in the bill. More importantly, the organizations again presented the positive data on the Voluntary Effort and again claimed that these data proved that a mandatory plan was unnecessary. Regarding the capital expenditures limitation, the lobbies pointed out that since $2.5 billion was clearly an arbitrary figure, adding another arbitrary $500,000 to the limit did not make it any better. In conclusion, each organization made it clear that it intended to continue its aggressive opposition to the bill.

The First Phase: Proponents in Control

The Commerce Committee scheduled deliberation on the cost containment bill to begin on May 22. Conflicts with other bills and an inability to obtain a quorum, a problem which was to plague the mark-up throughout, insured that progress was painfully slow. The resultant lack of momentum was disquieting to supporters of the bill since the decision to obtain approval in the Commerce Committee before attempting to do so in the Ways and Means Committee was taken because it was felt that Commerce presented an easier route for the bill.[7] It had been hoped that expeditious approval in the Commerce Committee would improve the chances of approval by the Ways and Means Committee, but the mark-up in Commerce was ultimately to last over eight weeks and the bill finally reported contained few similarities to the administration's original proposal.

As the committee began its consideration of the bill, it was clear that little consensus existed. Preliminary vote counts indicated that about 17 members were in favor of something like the Rogers proposal, about 20 members were generally opposed to any mandatory plan, and about 6 were undecided.[8] Vigorous lobbying ensued, therefore, as both sides of the controversy attempted to gain the 22 votes needed to assure a majority in the committee. The president wrote a letter to each member calling the bill "the most important immediate step" the country could take to hold down "intolerable" health costs, and a "top priority" to hold down inflation.[9] More importantly, the president telephoned the undecided members to urge a favorable vote for the Rogers proposal.

Meanwhile lobbyists for organized labor were at work opposing the bill because of their concerns about the effect the Voluntary Effort might have on the wage levels of hospital workers. Their success can be measured by the fact that they were able to keep a small group of liberal committee members uncommitted until those concerns were mitigated. More important to the final outcome of the controversy was that the provider lobbies were able to form a solid coalition against the bill whose strength never fell much below 20 members. With the support and leadership of Representatives Santini (D.-Nev.) and Broyhill (R.-N.C.), provider groups held a series of meetings in which they carefully mapped out their strategy and worked out their alternative proposal, the Santini amendment. In essence the committee's consideration of H.R. 6575 became an effort by the administration to wean away some of the support for the provider-backed coalition, while the coalition struggled to gain the one or two votes needed for a majority.

The first test of the relative strengths of these efforts occurred June 7 on a motion of Representative Gammage (D.-Texas) to recommit the bill to subcommittee. This delaying tactic failed on a 16 to 24 vote but the administration and its supporters could not be entirely happy with the result since two liberals, Waxman (D.-Calif.) and Eckhardt (D.-Texas), joined the committee conservatives in voting for recommittal. Moreover, several of those voting against recommittal announced that their vote did not mean that they supported the bill but that they believed the time had come to stop delaying and to vote cost containment up or down.

A far more important test of the opposing coalitions occurred on the provider-backed alternative, the Santini amendment. The amendment proposed to delete from Title I of the bill all references to the standby mandatory cost containment program, leaving in its place statutory recognition of the Voluntary Effort's goals and the study commission proposed by Rogers. In a "Dear Colleague" letter distributed before the vote, Republican opposition leader Broyhill and Representative Madigan (R.-Ill.) explained that they believed the "comprehensive effort the health care industry has made ... should be given a chance ... rather than imposing an inequitable system,"[10] while a letter from Santini recounted the reported impact of the voluntary program and reiterated the American Hospital Association's contention that "stand-by controls are inherently inflationary as hospitals would fear the imposition of a cap and would try to increase their base revenues up to the maximum level."[11] The debate on the amendment was less polite as highlighted by Santini's references to the many transformations the bill had undergone as it progressed from the administration's proposal to the Rogers substitute and by his characterization of the two versions as "turkey one" and "turkey two." He was admonished by Chairman Harley Staggers (D.-W.Va.) that such terms were not in keeping with the dignity of the committee. Rogers responded by terming Santini's proposal a "sham" and by forcefully claiming that nine states had been able to institute a cost containment program, leaving the implication that the committee did not have the courage to do what those states had been able to do.

Ultimately, the amendment failed on a 20 to 22 vote with cost containment opponent Madigan failing to cast a vote. Again, even though labor supporters Waxman and Eckhardt had voted against Santini, cost containment proponents could not have been entirely pleased since it was clear that the opponents' coalition was holding firm. The opposing coalitions and the closeness of the division in the committee were now clearly defined; the question was whether the proponents' coalition could retain its thin majority in light of the difficulties in meeting the conflicting demands of its liberal and conservative members. In retrospect, the most important of these problems was that Health Subcommittee ranking minority member Carter was the only Republican who did not vote in favor of the Santini amendment, leaving him isolated from his minority colleagues. The emergence of Broyhill as the Republican leader denied Carter his normal leadership role on health legislation, which must have been disquieting to Carter. Most importantly, the close division in the committee and the solid opposition of Republicans under Broyhill's leadership subjected Representative Carter to strong pressure by both provider lobbyists and his minority colleagues to change his position. Nevertheless, disconcerting as his position may have been, at this point Carter still appeared to be strongly supporting the Rogers substitute.

Cost containment supporters took several steps to solidify support for their position, the most important of which was an amendment proposed by Eckhardt of Texas reflecting organized labor's concerns about the effect of the Voluntary Effort on hospital workers' wages. In what has been termed an attempt to "buy the left,"[12] the amendment proposed to exclude the wages of nonsupervisory wage costs from the calculations of whether or not the voluntary goals had been met, thus mandating that the cost reductions necessary if hospitals were to stave off the imposition of mandatory controls must occur in the nonwage and supervisory wage costs of hospitals. Rogers had argued against special treatment for labor in negotiations with the administration, organized labor, and congressional labor supporters,[13] but the clear need to hold the votes of labor's supporters on the committee caused his criticism of the Eckhardt amendment to be relatively muted. Unfortunately, it appeared that Rogers's need to provide an opening to the left may have caused Carter, his only supporter on the right, to waver. Carter led the debate against the amendment, making essentially the same points that had been included in the Senate Human Resources Committee minority views on the issue,[14] claiming that "the available data [did] not support the contention" that the amendment was needed.[15] However, a majority did not agree and the amendment carried on a 15 to 12 vote.

The acceptance of the Eckhardt amendment by the committee led other members to propose two pass-throughs of their own. The first, offered by Representative Gammage, proposed to pass through all increased unit costs for energy; the second, offered by Representative David Stockman (R.-Mich.) proposed to pass through all increased costs for malpractice. Although the two amendments were narrowly defeated 19 to 20 and 19 to 21, respectively, the irony of providing pass-throughs for some costs and not for others was not lost on the committee, with Representative Wirth (D.-Colo.) noting that he hoped that the "mischief that was just raised here reflects the nonsense of adding pass-throughs."[16]

As the mark-up stretched into its second and third weeks, deliberation in the committee continued in the same fashion with opponents attempting to weaken the bill and proponents attempting to broaden their coalition through specific amendments designed to deal with an individual member's particular concerns. Broyhill attempted to give Congress a one-house veto over imposition of the mandatory cost containment program if the Voluntary Effort failed, but again his coalition was only able to muster 20 votes to 21 for the other side. Proponents accepted and supported an amendment offered by Representative Joe Skubitz (R.-Kan.) which effectively exempted all small rural hospitals from mandatory controls, the passage of which led Skubitz to indicate that he would support the bill on final passage. In a similar vein, the committee accepted an amendment proposed by Wirth to exempt from the mandatory controls any state which on its own had met the voluntary goals even if the national effort had failed.

The committee also accepted an amendment proposed by Madigan which provided that the maximum percentage increase allowed under the voluntary program would be increased or decreased as the GNP deflator increased or decreased as compared to the GNP deflator for 1977. However, the next day the amendment was withdrawn by unanimous consent and another Madigan amendment was accepted in its place which set the base year for mandatory controls at 1977 and guaranteed every hospital a transitional increase between 1977 and the start of mandatory controls equal to the voluntary program's goal. This curious action occurred because the first amendment tended to maintain the status quo relationship between the rate of increase in hospital costs and inflation in the rest of the economy, a relationship which cost containment supporters clearly wanted to change. On the other hand, the second amendment actually strengthened the Rogers substitute and the Voluntary Effort since by freezing the base year to a time before the Voluntary Effort started, it removed any incentive for hospitals to raise their revenue in anticipation of mandatory controls. Furthermore, the Rogers substitute proposed that between the base year and the first year of mandatory controls, hospitals would have only their actual inflation recognized. Under the

Madigan proposal, each hospital would be allowed increases equal to the Voluntary Effort's goals which meant that the lower cost hospitals, those whose inflation was less than the goals, would receive extra revenue when and if mandatory controls were imposed. Substitution of the second amendment for the first occurred because the problems with the first proposal were not immediately apparent to proponents of the bill. The second amendment was actually more important to the supporters of the Voluntary Effort because it was thought to provide a clear incentive to hospitals to bring their rate of increase below the goals, an action which in concert would stave off mandatory controls. For these reasons, it was in both groups' best interest for proponents to offer support for Madigan's second amendment if he would withdraw the first, and for his supporters to agree. It is important to point out that the members of the Santini-Broyhill coalition most likely would have never agreed to give up on an amendment which they had already won if they had been able to find the votes necessary to overcome cost containment supporters' active opposition on the second and more important amendment. However, their ability to influence events was about to take a turn for the better.

The Second Phase: Opponents Gaining Control

On the morning of June 21, Representative Carter turned to Chairman Staggers and asked to be recognized, indicating that he had a statement to make:

> I have worked very hard on this legislation—and I continue to support its goals. However, over the last few weeks I feel that our position has been compromised. First, the Voluntary Effort is no longer voluntary. There is a forced pass-through for nonsupervisory labor and not for other employees in the hospital. Second, it is my fear that the three billion dollar cap on capital expenditures is too small. However, this cap *would not apply* to the construction of a particular veterans hospital, since it is not included under this legislation. Moreover, the present attitude of the Administration in its attack on certain professionals cools my ardor for this legislation.
>
> While we all realize that the goal of this bill may be well-intentioned, the feasibility of constraining one segment of the economy while letting others run wildly verges on the impossible. If we're going to have a pass-through for labor, well then, we should have a pass-through for nonlabor costs as well.
>
> Mr. Chairman, I've never been a part of such bargaining under one Administration as has occurred with this legislation. These events remind me of an earlier occasion when I was told of a project that would have been helpful to two counties in my district, and that my vote was needed on a particular bill. To this I responded: 'You can take the project and do what you want with it, I'm going to vote as I please.'

Mr. Chairman, the unusual wheeling and dealing on this legislation has turned me off, so for what it may be worth, I reserve the right to vote as I feel is right.[17]

That Carter had reached a point at which he could no longer support the bill is perhaps not surprising, in consideration of his conservative stance and his position as a physician. Nevertheless, Carter had remained in support of the bill until a combination of events caused him to disassociate himself from it. First, HEW Secretary Califano had announced on June 20 that he was signing a notice of intent to "propose a regulation that will prohibit doctors, hospital administrators, and others with a strong financial stake in the health care industry . . . from dominating the governing boards of organizations that process and pay . . . bills for Medicare and Medicaid,"[18] which mainly would affect Blue Cross/Blue Shield. Second, a draft of the Health Maintenance Organization Amendments of 1978 had proposed to delete from the law the requirement of Section 1303(b)(1)(B) of the Public Health Service Act that organizations which intend to conduct a survey of the feasibility of establishing an HMO shall so notify the local medical societies. These were the "attacks on certain professionals" which cooled Carter's ardor.

Carter was also alluding to the fact that consideration of the cost containment bill had been marred by charges that the administration had bought favorable votes in exchange for certain favors. The most widely discussed charge was that the administration had dropped its opposition to a new Veterans Administration hospital in Camden, New Jersey in exchange for a favorable vote from Representative James Florio (D.-N.J.). The House Appropriations Committee had already indicated that it would approve the hospital for Camden at this time, but the allegation stuck. Moreover, rumors were being circulated that charged that votes were being "bought" with water projects, delayed military base closings, and promises of primary-time visits to congressional districts by prominent administration officials.[19]

However, it is not completely certain that Representative Carter's change of position followed directly from the charges that he made in his statement. It must also be pointed out that Carter was being lobbied heavily by the AMA, his natural constituency, as well as by hospital administrators in his district. Furthermore, his position on cost containment had isolated him from his minority colleagues, as well as removing him from his traditional conservative stance in opposition to increased federal regulation. For these reasons, it is equally likely to conclude that although Carter's concern about escalating hospital costs was genuine enough to cause him to support the bill in its early stages, the combination of his own beliefs plus pervasive lobbying by providers and his colleagues caused Carter to return to a position which he may have preferred all along.

With Carter apparently disgruntled and his position unclear, the committee moved to consider the next major effort by the opponents' coalition to weaken the bill substantially. An amendment by Stockman proposed to remove the disincentives towards increasing admissions and incentives towards decreasing admissions contained in the original bill. Instead of allowing hospitals only 50 percent of the average per admission revenue for increases within a specified range over the base year as did the original bill, Stockman proposed to increase revenue by 100 percent of that average amount for each increased admission. In the case of decreases, the original bill proposed to hold revenue constant if admissions dropped less than 6 percent; from 6 percent to 15 percent, the bill proposed to decrease revenue by an amount equal to 50 percent of average per admission revenue. In contrast, the Stockman amendment proposed a decrease equal to 75 percent of average per admission revenue as soon as the number of admissions dropped below the base year level, but only in so far as admissions dropped less than 5 percent. After that point, revenue would decrease by 100 percent of the average per admission revenue.

Stockman had provided the committee with a great deal of material in support of his position against the legislation and particularly in support of his amendment.[20] In three "Dear Colleague" letters, one of which contained 28 pages, Stockman argued that the rising number of inputs, rather than rising prices, was the driving force behind hospital inflation and that there was a direct connection between these rising inputs and a better quality of medical care. He had further argued that an increasing elderly population was causing the complexity of hospital case mix to increase, and that arbitrary limits on revenue would affect the older portion of the population. Finally, he had argued that the admission adjustments contained in the bill would subject hospitals to a revenue limit below the rate of inflation for the economy as a whole if their admissions were rising.

There was a great deal of information which Stockman did not mention, much of it related to the research cited earlier in this book. There would be little argument that rising inputs rather than rising prices are the more important factors explaining inflation in hospital care expenditures. Where argument would occur is on Stockman's contention that there was not enough proof to indicate that much of the increase in inputs was unnecessary or duplicative. There would also be argument as to whether the *continued* rapid increases in hospital costs could be attributed to increases in the elderly population and facilitation of their access to medical care. As was pointed out in Chapter 3, dramatic increases in inputs have occurred across the entire spectrum of case complexity and patient age groups; clearly many of those cannot be attributed to medical care for the elderly.

Nevertheless, Stockman's basic argument rested on the point that the cost containment bill involved the use of arbitrary limits which may or may not have achieved the desired results. He was willing to concede that some input increases or admission increases were unnecessary, but he was not willing to concede that there was enough "slack" in the system to absorb the impact of the revenue limits. Stockman's most telling point was that the marginal cost assumptions involved in the admission load formula were based on three studies conducted by P. Feldstein,[21] Lave and Lave,[22] and by M. Feldstein[23] that were over a decade old and which arrived at dissimilar conclusions. The three studies found that marginal costs ranged from 21 to 74 percent of average costs, rather than the 50 percent assumption proposed by the administration.

Debate on the Stockman amendment was relatively brief, probably because by this point in the mark-up, it seemed to be more of a question of who proposed an amendment than of the merits of the issue. Moreover, Rogers and his supporters were no doubt reasonably certain that they had the votes to turn back Stockman. Rogers did refer to the ability of hospital administrators to increase admissions if such action were necessary to increase revenue, the problem with which the admission load formula was designed to deal, and cited a Las Vegas hospital which was offering patients a chance to win a vacation if they checked into the hospital the weekend before their scheduled surgery.[24] Moss also entered into the debate, citing the evidence on unnecessary surgery gathered by his Subcommittee on Oversight and Investigations.

As the committee's clerk called the roll on the Stockman amendment, it was clear to staff members keeping a running tally that the vote was proceeding similarly to most of the previous votes. It appeared as if all of the Republicans except Carter plus the eight Democrats in the Santini-Broyhill coalition would vote for Stockman's amendment. The first surprise was that Democrat Albert Gore (D.-Tenn.) voted with Stockman, a move which he later attributed to his concerns about the lack of medical care in his Appalachian district.[25] Nevertheless, one member of the coalition was not available to vote and had not filed a proxy with the committee, so it still appeared as if the amendment would fail by one vote. (A proxy is a notice which allows a member to cast a vote for an absent colleague.) At a pause in the vote, Carter turned to the chair and asked how he was recorded. The clerk noted that he was recorded as voting "no;" Carter thought for a moment, and then said to the clerk, "off no, on aye." The Stockman amendment was agreed to on a 21 to 20 vote; the Santini-Broyhill coalition had won its first victory because Carter seemingly had decided that he was not going to vote to sustain the administration's position against all of the other Republicans if the administration was going to wheel and deal for votes and engage in what Carter regarded as gratuitous attacks on the medical profession.

Preliminary estimates by the Congressional Budget Office and by HEW indicated that the Stockman amendment might wipe out all of the savings associated with the original bill. Thus, Rogers and the administration moved quickly in an attempt to overturn the amendment.[26] A new compromise admission load formula was devised which was a great deal more lenient than the first, and was packaged into a new amendment to be offered by Representative Richardson Preyer (D.-N.C.). The administration sent Health Care Financing Administrator Robert Derzon up to the Hill to lobby key members in favor of the Preyer amendment. Finally, a letter was sent to all members of the committee laying out the arguments against the Stockman amendment.[27] The letter pointed out the fear shared by many that revenue limits provided an incentive to hospitals to increase admissions in the absence of any volume controls, a point substantiated by experience with the Economic Stabilization Program and with the Connecticut Rate Review Commission. The letter further noted that Stockman had underestimated the actual allowable increase in per admission revenues under the original bill since Stockman had not properly adjusted for the effects of increasing admissions in previous years. Most important, the letter highlighted Stockman's omission of the fact that a hospital would always receive an increase in *total* revenue even though the admission load formula might have been causing allowable revenue *per admission* to increase at a slower rate. The lack of clarity on this last point in the committee had enhanced Stockman's argument that the admission load formula would cause hospital revenue to increase at a rate less than that of the rest of the economy.

An inability to insure a quorum and the hiatus caused by the July 4 congressional recess gave both sides a great deal of time to prepare for the consideration of the Preyer amendment. It was clear that Rogers and his supporters needed to convince Carter or Gore, and possibly both, to change their position on the admission formula, and a great deal of effort was expended in trying to do so. That effort, though, was not successful, leaving Rogers with insufficient votes to obtain approval of the Preyer amendment. For that reason the Preyer amendment was withdrawn, and the Stockman amendment was left in place.

Withdrawal of the Preyer amendment was a watershed for cost containment in the House because prospects for committee approval of the standby mandatory control plan only worsened after this point. The committee turned down a proposal of Representative Anthony Toby Moffett (D.-Conn.) to require physicians to accept assignment of Medicare claims insuring, in effect, that physicians would receive no more for Medicare claims than the government was willing to pay them. The failure of the amendment caused a threat by Moffett to vote against the bill on final passage. Representative Satterfield's amendment to delete the $3 billion capital expenditures limit was rejected by the committee, but Satterfield's proposal raised an entirely new set of objections on which the committee had not focused before this point. This led the committee to agree with Carter's proposal to raise the limit to $4 billion, the need for which Carter had alluded to in his earlier statement.

The Third Phase: Showdown

Nevertheless, at that point it still looked as if the committee would approve a bill by a narrow margin, even if the reported bill had lost most of its teeth. Representatives Carter and Skubitz had indicated in public that they would vote for the bill on final passage, and it appeared that Moffett would go along. It looked as if Rogers could command 23 votes, one more than absolutely needed, to get the bill through. What was not generally known, however, was that Carter had instructed the Health Subcommittee's minority staff to write a new amendment which would incorporate: (1) the Santini amendment's deletion of mandatory controls; (2) the Rogers proposal for a monitoring and study commission; (3) Carter's proposal for support of state cost containment programs; and (4) the provisions from the Health Subcommittee's reported bill (H.R. 9717) providing for swing beds for rural hospitals, coordinated audits for Medicare and Medicaid, and a study of the impact of federal regulation on hospital costs. Moreover, Representative Carter had instructed the staff to inform the members of the Santini-Broyhill coalition of his plans in order to garner support for a new proposal of his. The result of such meetings was that it was decided that Broyhill should introduce the amendment and that Carter would support it.

On July 18, Broyhill proposed the amendment with very little debate; most of the arguments had previously been heard. Each side of the controversy had 20 votes with 3 undecided. They were Skubitz, unsure because of concern that a "yes" vote on Broyhill might be construed as bending his earlier promise to Rogers; Matthew J. Rinaldo, (R.-N.J.) who had not attended many of the committee's sessions and whose position was not clear; and Martin A. Russo (D.-Ill.) who it was rumored had requested information about the new Broyhill amendment in advance. The vote proceeded on the predictable lines of many of its predecessors until Russo's name was called. When Russo voted "aye," immediate consternation erupted in the committee room and Rogers was propelled out of his seat to try to convince Russo to change before the vote was over. As the clerk called the names of the Republicans, Skubitz voted "aye" and Rinaldo voted "no," thus leaving Russo's vote as the deciding one in a 22 to 21 victory for the opponents of cost containment and finally defeating the idea of federal action at this time to stem the rising costs of hospital care. In its place, the committee had left: (1) the providers' Voluntary Effort; (2) federal funding for states to attempt to contain costs on their own; and (3) a $4 billion cap applicable only to capital expenditures on which the country had spent about $1 billion in 1977.

The committee then perfunctorily voted to report what remained of the bill to the House with Rogers barely concealing his anger and vowing an attempt to recreate a tougher bill when it reached the floor of the House. A major question which remained in most observers' minds was why Russo had changed his position, and it must be kept in mind that Russo had voted against the original Santini amendment. Although several newspaper columnists have castigated Russo for changing his vote, it is not at all clear why he did so.[28] There was one event occurring during the mark-up which may have influenced Russo's, and perhaps to some extent Carter's, change of position. Early in July, Chairman Rogers announced that he would not be running for reelection in November, an announcement that literally caught all but a few of his close associates by surprise. A retiring member is obviously not going to return next year to wield whatever power he may have gained, and the retirement of "Mr. Health" may have provided cost containment critics the freedom of movement to oppose Rogers's position.

However, although the cost containment bill was close to being defeated as a result of the Commerce Committee's actions, there were still a few avenues open to cost containment supporters. The first was an attempt to get Ways and Means to pass a bill like the original Rogers substitute, but this was thought to be highly unlikely since the Ways and Means Health Subcommittee had reported out a similar bill with only a one-vote margin. It should be remembered that one of the reasons the Commerce Committee had taken up the bill first was because it was thought that passage by the Commerce Committee would provide enough momentum to get the bill through a more antagonistic Ways and Means Committee. The futility of attempting to obtain approval from Ways and Means of a strong bill was confirmed when a Ways and Means spokesman announced that there was little possibility that Ways and Means would act on the Rostenkowski compromise bill reported by his Subcommittee on Health early in February. The spokesman pointed out that Ways and Means expected to concentrate its efforts on tax legislation until September, and the cost containment bill would not come up after that "unless it were absolutely guaranteed that [the committee] would not be in a protracted war" over it.[29] In consideration of the "war" which had occurred in the Commerce Committee over the bill, there was little likelihood that a similar struggle could be avoided in Ways and Means.

A more realistic st. ategy was an attempt to obtain approval in the Senate for some kind of cost containment bill, although at that point that also appeared highly unlikely. The Senate Human Resources Committee had approved a bill very similar to the administration's over a year before, but that bill could not be brought to the floor until it was approved by Senator Talmadge's Health Subcommittee and its parent, the full Finance Committee. Talmadge had not taken up the administration's bill, but had instead begun marking-up his Medicare-Medicaid Administrative Reform Act (S. 1470) on June 21.

Senate Action

When the Finance Committee met in early August to consider S. 1470, as reported by the committee's Subcommittee on Health, a new administration strategy to obtain approval of the stalled legislation became apparent. Instead of retiring in defeat, the administration had used the short hiatus between the setback in the Commerce Committee and the beginning of consideration of the Talmadge bill by the Finance Committee to design a new compromise proposal. Under the sponsorship of Senator Gaylord Nelson (D.-Wisc.), the new proposal incorporated elements of the Talmadge bill and the administration's bill as well as the Rostenkowski/Voluntary Effort compromise bill rejected by the Commerce Committee. In this way the outlines of the final debate in the 95th Congress on controlling hospital costs were drawn—a reimbursement reform bill with relatively modest cost savings which ultimately could apply mandatory revenue restrictions to almost every hospital.

The Talmadge Bill (S. 1470)

The version of S. 1470 considered by the Finance Committee was not much different from the bill originally proposed by Talmadge (see Chapter 7). The bill proposed to classify hospitals in groups by bed size, location (rural versus urban), type of hospital (teaching versus nonteaching), and other categories which HEW later found to be appropriate. A per diem routine operating cost target rate would be calculated for each hospital by calculating an average per diem routine operating cost by group, and then adjusting the group average for each hospital to reflect prevailing wage rates in the hospital's area. A hospital whose actual routine operating costs exceeded the target rate would be paid its actual costs up to a ceiling of 115 percent of the target rate for the relevant group; hospitals whose costs were below the target rate would be able to retain 50 percent of the difference between their actual costs and the target, up to a maximum of 5 percent of the target rate.

As a hospital cost containment proposal, this new reimbursement system proposed by Talmadge clearly had its limitations. First, the bonuses and limitations proposed would apply only to Medicare and Medicaid or about 41 percent of total hospital costs.[30] Second, the system would apply only to certain routine operating costs (routine nursing, administrative, maintenance, supply, and food costs), but would exclude the routine operating costs associated with the costs of capital, education and training programs, malpractice insurance, energy, and all ancillary services. These costs amount to only about 40 percent of total hospital costs, with the net result, HEW estimated, that the Talmadge bill would apply to less than 20 percent of all hospital costs.[31] A further problem was that in calculating the average for each group in the second and succeeding years of the program, HEW was directed to count 50 percent of the amount of any hospital's costs in excess of 115 percent of the target rate. This would mean that unreasonably high costs for hospitals within a group would raise the following year's average. Also, the new reimbursement system might have caused greater responsibility for hospital revenue to be shifted to other payers, as limits were applied to Medicare and Medicaid. Perhaps most importantly, the limitations on reimbursement proposed by the bill were to be applied on a per diem basis and, as the research cited in Chapter 4 has demonstrated, controls on reimbursement applied on a per diem basis bring with them the risk that hospitals may inappropriately raise their average length of stay in an attempt to avoid the effects of the controls.

On the positive side, the Talmadge bill encompassed the first attempt to put reasonable limits on the present open-ended retrospective reimbursement system. Although the grouping methodology proposed was relatively limited, especially when compared to grouping methodologies used in some states, the bill provided a mechanism for improving the system by granting to HEW open-ended authority to add other appropriate classification variables. The bill also established a Health Facilities Cost Commission to "monitor and study all aspects of the cost reimbursement program and propose such changes and refinements as it found appropriate."[32] The commission specifically was directed to study the possible application of the new system to other hospital costs such as ancillary service costs, an action which ultimately could lead to correction of the greatest weakness of the proposal, its limited application.

It should also be pointed out that the bill proposed several other kinds of changes designed to improve the Medicare and Medicaid programs. Similar to the House Commerce Committee bill, the Finance Committee proposed to allow small rural hospitals to be reimbursed for nursing home care services when they used their acute-care beds as long-term care beds. The bill also would have mandated common audits for Medicare and Medicaid, and would have removed existing restrictions on the use of home care services by Medicare recipients. Further proposals were designed to encourage physicians to accept assignment of Medicare claims, and thus receive their entire reimbursement directly from Medicare; other provisions proposed to alter physician reimbursement schedules to encourage ambulatory surgery and the establishment of physician's practices in medically underserved areas.

One of the most interesting provisions of the Finance Committee bill was a proposal to include in payments to short-term hospitals reimbursement for increased operating costs and, for nonprofit hospitals only, increased capital costs associated with the closing down or conversion to approved uses of underutilized beds or services. Under this provision the nonprofit hospitals could continue to receive reimbursement for depreciation or interest on debt associated with the closed beds; if an entire hospital were closed, payment would continue until any debt was repaid. The most interesting aspect of this proposal is that it would be capable of providing incentives, and payments, for the closure of excess capacity without requiring authorization of a new categorical program as had the excess capacity buy-out program in the House Commerce bill.

In presenting this bill to the Senate, Senator Talmadge emphasized its modest dimensions. He characterized the bill as making "orderly modifications in various aspects of physician reimbursement, long-term care, and the general provisions of Medicare and Medicaid."[33] The senator went to some length to point out that the bill was "not a system for controlling all hospital costs," but was a bill "to change the way Medicare and Medicaid reimburse hospitals."[34] Most importantly, he stated that the "bill is not the Government in its role as regulator—it is the Government in its role as a purchaser of hospital care, the Government as a prudent buyer."[35]

The Nelson Amendment

In contrast, the administration and its supporters clearly felt that reforms on federal reimbursement were not sufficient. They believed that inflation in hospital costs was so severe that the government must act in its role of regulator, and President Carter threatened to veto the Talmadge bill if the Congress passed it without provisions which limited total hospital spending as the administration had originally proposed.[36] The vehicle developed by the administration and its supporters to obtain approval of hospital revenue limitations was the amendment proposed by Senator Nelson for inclusion in S. 1470.

The Nelson amendment included something from almost every hospital cost containment bill proposed in the 95th Congress. First it incorporated the new system for reimbursement of routine operating costs from the Talmadge bill but with several modifications. As noted, the original Talmadge bill required HEW to include in its calculation of group averages for the second and succeeding years of the program, 50 percent of the amount by which each hospital's costs were in excess of the 115 percent limitation; the Nelson amendment disregarded all amounts in excess of the limitation. The amendment placed further restrictions on inflation in federal reimbursement by limiting annual routine operating cost increases to 1.5 times the rate of increase in a market basket of goods and services normally purchased by a hospital. The amendment included this limitation because under the original Talmadge bill, according to Senator Nelson, a hospital which had been operating at 80 percent of the target rate could increase its routine operating costs up to 115 percent of the rate, an increase of nearly 50 percent, without any penalty. The Nelson amendment further modified the proposed changes in reimbursement by allowing the secretary of HEW to implement changes proposed by the Health Facilities Cost Commission to extend the system beyond its original limited scope without returning to Congress for further legislative authority.

The Nelson amendment went far beyond simply modifying the basic Talmadge reimbursement reforms by proposing to recognize the goals of the Voluntary Effort as originally proposed by Rostenkowski, and by establishing a system of standby mandatory controls as proposed by the administration and modified by the Kennedy, Rogers, and Rostenkowski subcommittees. The amendment did not include any of the limitations on capital expenditures originally proposed in Title II of the administration bill, nor did it include the Commerce Committee's proposal to reduce excess capacity.

As is reasonable to expect, the combination of several different proposals plus efforts to answer various criticisms of earlier versions of those proposals (such as organized labor's concerns about the impact of the program on hospital workers' wages) caused the Nelson amendment to be a very complex piece of legislation. This point is demonstrated by the following illustration which describes the Nelson amendment in terms of its impact on a hypothetical hospital:

Community Hospital is a hypothetical 300-bed acute care hospital that averages about 12,000 admissions per year. This illustration assumes passage of Section 2 of the Talmadge bill, with the Nelson amendment, in October of 1978.

Prior to January 1, 1979, Community Hospital would report its expenses for each calendar quarter of 1976, 1977, and the first three quarters of 1978. It would continue to file quarterly reports for each succeeding quarter within 60 days of the close of the quarter. These reports would also indicate the amount of increase in expense arising for increases in the average hourly wage rates for non-supervisory employees.

For purposes of this example, assume that Community Hospital reports the following data:

1976	spending:	$20 million
1977	spending:	23 million
1978	spending:	26 million

In addition it reports that $1 million of the increase in both 1977 and 1978 resulted from increased wage rates.

In March of 1979 the Health Care Financing Administration (HEW) would add the expenses of Community Hospital with the expenses of all other reporting hospitals, disregarding the amounts arising from increased wage rates for nonsupervisory employees. For purposes of this example, assume that the increase nationally and in the state are as follows:

	State	Nation
1977..............	16%	16%
1978..............	13%	13%

Since the voluntary goal is a 2 percent reduction in 1978, and the hospitals nationally dropped from 16 percent to 13 percent (a 3 percent reduction), the voluntary goal was met and no further controls are triggered anywhere in the nation.

HEW Implements the Talmadge Reforms

At the same time (during March of 1979) the secretary of HEW would announce the Medicare and Medicaid routine operating cost target rates for each hospital as computed under the Talmadge bill. Assume that for hospitals with 300 beds in Community Hospital's area, the target based on average costs among similar hospitals is $100 per day starting January 1, 1980. Community Hospital enters that accounting year knowing that routine operating expenses in excess of $115 per day will be disallowed by Medicare and Medicaid, and that expenses of less than $100 per day will earn the hospital bonus payments.

The Voluntary Effort Fails

All hospitals would continue to report quarterly data during 1979 in order to allow for continued monitoring of the voluntary goals. In March, 1980, HEW would again add all reported expenses from Community Hospital and all other reporting hospitals (excluding expenses arising from increased wage rates). Assume that the increase during 1979 was 13 percent nationally and 13 percent in Community Hospital's state (taking into account the state's increased population). Since the national voluntary goal is a rate of increase of 12 percent, the secretary of HEW would announce that the voluntary goal has been exceeded both nationally and in Community Hospital's state. Standby controls would be effective January 1, 1980. . . .

At the same time, the secretary would announce two sets of data necessary to implement the standby controls:

The rate of increase in wages of service workers in each hospital's locality for the most recent two year period for which data are available.

The rate of increase in a market basket index reflecting nonlabor purchases of hospitals. This index would be derived from appropriate components of the CPI and WPI weighted to reflect hospital purchases.

For purposes of this illustration, assume that wages increased by 9 percent in Community Hospital's area and that the price index increased by 8 percent.

Standby Limits Implemented

The Medicare Intermediary for Community Hospital would review its estimate of 1980 costs to assure against payments in excess of the limits. Assume that it estimates:

Twelve thousand admissions.

Routine costs comprise one-third of costs and nonroutine, non-labor costs and nonroutine labor costs each comprise one-third.

Routine operating costs were $100 per day in the previous year.

A pay raise will increase the average hourly wage rate for non-supervisory employees by 12 percent and such wages will constitute 40 percent of Community Hospital's costs.

Based on these estimates, the intermediary would compute the standby limit on reimbursement per inpatient admission according to the following steps:

1. Percentage by which routine costs can increase over the prior accounting year without being disallowed:

$$\frac{\$115 - \$100}{\$100} = .15$$

2. Reduced by excess over 1½ times the "market basket" index used in setting target rates under the Talmadge bill (assume 8%):

.15 − .03 = .12 (8% times 1.5 = 12%. 15% computed under step one is in excess of 12% by 3%)

3. Multiply by portion of costs representing routine operating costs:

$$.12 \times \frac{1}{3} = .04$$

4. Add the product of the increase in area wages (9%) times the portion of nonroutine labor costs (one-third):

$$.04 + (.09 \times \frac{1}{3}) = .07$$

5. Add the product of the increase in the 'market basket' index of nonlabor hospital prices (8%) times the portion those costs constitute of total costs (one-third):

$$.07 + (.08 \times \frac{1}{3}) = .0966$$

6. Subtract the product of the percentage by which Community Hospital was in excess of the voluntary goal for 1979 (assume that it experienced a 13% increase) times the portion of hospital expense which does not arise from regular wages of nonsupervisory employees (60%):

$$.0966 - (.13 - .12)(.6) = .0906$$

7. Multiply by the portion of costs represented by costs other than the regular wages of nonsupervisory employees:

$$.0906 \times .6 = .05436$$

8. Add the product of the rate increase in the regular wages of nonsupervisory employees times the proportion of total costs arising from such wages (40%):

$$.05436 + (.12 \times .4) = .10236$$

The intermediary would inform the hospital that Medicare payment per admission in 1980 cannot exceed such payments in 1979 by more than 10.236 percent. In addition, the intermediary would notify the state Medicaid agency, all other third party payers paying on the basis of costs, and the hospital in computing its charges, that such amounts cannot exceed the limits. If they do exceed the limits, they would be subject to an excise tax.[37]

The most interesting thing about the Nelson amendment is the manner in which it incorporated many of the ideas which had been proposed by members of the three other committees which had already considered the hospital cost containment bill. Besides building upon the Talmadge and Rostenkowski proposals, the amendment also required the Voluntary Effort to meet its proposed goals in terms of nonwage costs as proposed in the House Commerce Committee by Congressmen Eckhardt (D.-Texas) and Waxman (D.-Calif.). It included the exemption from mandatory controls for hospitals in a state which by itself met the voluntary goals proposed by Congressman Wirth (D.-Colo.). Also included was the idea of tying the overall mandatory limit to a market basket index of hospital goods and services, as originally proposed by Congressman Carter in his cost containment bill. The bill also incorporated the exemption from mandatory controls for states which had their own cost containment programs, but included the requirement that new state programs provide for a nonsupervisory wage pass-through, a provision which was part of the bill approved by the Kennedy subcommittee.

Nevertheless, even though the Nelson amendment incorporated the proposals of many of those involved in the cost containment debate, the Finance Committee chose on a 7 to 11 vote not to accept it and instead sent the Talmadge bill to the Senate floor.

It was still possible, however, to obtain Senate approval of a stronger cost containment bill by proposing Nelson's amendment on the Senate floor. Nelson's announcement that he intended to do so was followed by Senator Kennedy's notice that he would offer Title I of the Human Resources Committee's approved mandatory cost containment plan as an amendment to Talmadge. Nevertheless, with the Senate postponing consideration of the Talmadge bill until after the Senate's Labor Day recess, it was difficult to see how agreement on a cost containment bill could be reached in the four weeks remaining in the 95th Congress. It should be kept in mind that even if Nelson or Kennedy were successful in securing agreement on either of their amendments, the bill still had to be voted on by the Senate and sent to the House. To expedite action on the bill, the Finance Committee had attached the reimbursement reform proposal to H.R. 5285, a minor bill already passed by the House. H.R. 5285 had proposed originally to amend the Tariff Schedules with respect to the treatment accorded to film, strips, sheets, and plates of certain plastics and rubber. The reason for adding the Talmadge bill to H.R. 5285 was that since the bill had already passed the House, when and if it passed the Senate, the bill could go immediately to a House-Senate Conference rather than waiting for a separate House vote on the issue. This could occur even though the Finance Committee had stricken all of the House-passed language relating to tariffs and inserted in its place only the committee version of the Talmadge bill.

The committee's decision to reject the Nelson amendment immediately led to a loud public argument between Senator Talmadge and HEW Secretary Califano. Califano complained that the savings from the Talmadge bill were miniscule compared with those associated with the Nelson amendment or the administration's proposal.[38] In this respect the secretary was on firm ground since it was estimated that the Talmadge bill would save only $500 million over the first five years,[39] while an estimated $55 to 60 billion would be saved under the administration's proposal[40] and an estimated $30 to 34 billion under the Nelson amendment[41] (although a later estimate by the Congressional Budget Office estimated savings from the Nelson amendment at $23.6 billion).[42] Talmadge responded by charging that Califano was comparing "apples and oranges" and that in so doing Califano had attacked the credibility and integrity of the Finance Committee.[43] Nevertheless, in obtaining approval of the plan on which he had worked for five years, Talmadge still faced the threat that President Carter would veto the bill if tougher cost containment measures were not included.

Further attacks on the Talmadge proposal were inherent in a briefing that the administration conducted for senators in the White House early in September. One of the most telling points included in the briefing document provided to senators and their staff was that the success of the Voluntary Effort, as demonstrated by a lower rate of increase in hospital expenses, was due mostly to actions of the *mandatory* programs operated in several states.[44] HEW had estimated that total inpatient hospital expenses rose 14.2 percent in 1977; in the 9 states with mandatory programs, the rate was only 12 percent while the 3 states with statutory voluntary programs experienced a 15.6 percent increase and the 39 states without any program (including the District of Columbia) experienced a 15.9 percent increase. Based upon this information, supporters of standby mandatory controls were able to claim that the Talmadge bill with its modest goals, and the Voluntary Effort without the threat of mandatory sanctions, were not sufficient.[45] Further evidence for their point of view came with the release of the Consumer Price Index for August which indicated that health care costs went up .9 percent in August while the hospital room and board component of the index rose 1.5 percent, an annual rate of 18 percent.[46]

Senate Floor Action

The last piece of the administration's cost containment strategy became clear upon Senator Kennedy's announcement that he would attempt to amend the Talmadge/Finance Committee bill with Title I of the Human Resources Committee bill approved over a year before. However, the debate was not to be a three-way struggle between Talmadge, Nelson, and Kennedy. Instead, it was clear that Kennedy and Nelson would work together in attempting first to obtain approval of the Human Resources bill; if that failed they would work together to pass Nelson's amendment. In fact, Nelson announced that he would vote for the Kennedy-backed bill and would offer his amendment on the floor only if that strategy failed.[47] It is hard to believe, however, that passage of the carefully drafted and complex Nelson amendment was not the ultimate goal of the administration forces. It is important to keep in mind that by offering first the Kennedy bill with its totally mandatory controls, the administration gave to the Nelson amendment an air of reasonable compromise with which it might not otherwise have been blessed.

On the other hand, obtaining time for consideration of the cost containment bill was no simple task even with its powerful backing. During the closing days of a congressional session, Congress often avoids bills expected to engender a great deal of controversy because of the large amount of time they consume. There was no question that a bill which pitted Senator Talmadge against Senators Kennedy and Nelson was one which would take up a great deal of time. An equally important obstacle was that Senate action on the bill would be futile if the House did not act, and of course the House had shown no signs that it planned to move forward; in fact, the opposite was anticipated. Finally, neither House had at this point acted on the two major issues of the 95th Congress, i.e., energy and the tax cut bill.

The first attempt to get the cost containment bill moving occurred just after Congress returned from its August recess, but the bill kept getting pushed back on the Senate's schedule. A serious effort was made on October 6 to attach the bill as an amendment to the tax bill, but a filibuster foiled the effort. Finally, with less than one week left in the 95th Congress, Senator Kennedy reportedly conferred with Senate Majority Leader Robert Byrd urging that the cost containment issue be considered.[48] On October 12 a bill concerning price supports for sugar was brought to the floor, and the Finance Committee bill, H.R. 5285, was introduced as an amendment to it. The Senate finally decided to set aside the sugar bill and consider H.R. 5285 alone.

The Senate debate on cost containment was not particularly different from all of the discussions which had already occurred in various forums, not surprisingly after months of debate on the subject.[49] Senator Nelson attacked the Talmadge bill, reciting the figures on inflation in hospital care and noting the small savings estimated under the Talmadge proposal. Senator Talmadge, backed by Senators Dole, Schweiker, and Curtis, criticized the administration, Kennedy, and Nelson proposals, noting the lack of specificity and selectiveness of a cap on hospital revenue, and pointing out the unknown impact of that cap on needed hospital services. Talmadge summed up his argument, stating, "While clearly—and perhaps brutally effective as a cost control device—[the bill] entails risks for the sick and disabled and their families that few Americans would wish to take."[50] Senator Schweiker reiterated the position he had taken earlier in subcommittee deliberations that the wage pass-throughs included in the proposals were unnecessary and highly inflationary in themselves. Kennedy countered by noting the success of the nine mandatory state programs in containing costs without any apparent decline in quality, while Nelson provided for the record a list of organizations in support of his amendment, including the Health Insurance Institute, the national associations representing cities, counties, state legislatures, and governors, as well as various organizations representing labor, health maintenance organizations, and other nonprovider health organizations. Senators Javits, Sasser, Riegle, Muskie, and others added their voices on behalf of Nelson.

The first test of the strength of the opposing sides came upon a motion by Senator Talmadge to table the Human Resources Committee version of the administration bill backed by Senator Kennedy. On this vote Talmadge prevailed 69 to 18 with 13 not voting. However, when Talmadge similarly moved to table the Nelson "compromise," the vote was 42 "ayes" to 47 "nays" with 11 not voting. The administration had finally won a vote on hospital cost containment with a little more than 72 hours remaining in the 95th Congress.

After the failure of the Talmadge motion to table the Nelson amendment, a motion by Senator Dole to provide for a legislative veto of the "triggering" of mandatory revenue controls should the Voluntary Effort fail was accepted by Nelson, even though Senators Kennedy and Brooke argued strongly against it. The move was curious because the Senate has traditionally opposed legislative vetoes, and had threatened to hold up a bill authorizing funds for the Federal Trade Commission if the House insisted on including such authority. A possible explanation for the acceptance of the Dole amendment is that immediately after Nelson stated that he was prepared to accept the amendment, Talmadge announced that he was "prepared to accept the *Nelson* amendment, as modified."[51] Thus, after a long debate on the relative merits of the Talmadge and administration approaches to hospital costs, the Nelson amendment was agreed to on a voice vote. The final and almost irrelevant vote passing H.R. 5285, as amended, was 64 to 22 with 14 not voting.

Conclusion

What kind of cost containment bill had the administration and its supporters bought with their many compromises? The bill contained the new Talmadge system for federal reimbursement of hospitals, a system which because of its relatively weak cost containment controls was almost irrelevant, since if the inflationary trends noted in August continued, causing the Voluntary Effort to fail, much more stringent mandatory controls would be imposed on all hospitals. The bill had further problems related to the triggering of the mandatory controls if the Voluntary Effort failed. The bill already exempted hospitals in states in which the voluntary goals were met. As a result of an amendment offered by Senator Richard Stone (D.-Fla.), the Senate also had agreed to exempt any individual *hospital* which met the voluntary goals. Aside from the administrative complexity of a program which controlled some hospitals and not others, even when hospitals in one group or the other might be just across the street from each other, there was the further problem of deciding just who *had* met the goals. Senator Schweiker perhaps best characterized the problem when he stated, "We are going to have to engage in a great number of statistical arguments about this hospital and that hospital. As soon as we put an amendment to exempt individual hospitals, I guarantee that every Senator's office is going to have dozens of hospitals coming into his office with a battery of lawyers to get exempted, and each Senator here is going to be arguing with or cajoling HEW about whether one of their hospitals back home is going to be covered or not."[52]

The inclusion of the individual hospital exemption and the acceptance of the legislative veto by the Senate says a great deal about administration strategy. There was very little chance that the House was going to act in the short time remaining; with less than three days left in the congressional session, the House had not considered either the energy or the tax bill. Considering that the House had to meet around the clock on October 14 and 15 to finish its consideration of those two major issues as well as a host of others, it appeared that the chance for convening of a Conference Committee and passage of a conference report in the House were very slim indeed. However, if the administration was going to bring up hospital cost containment in the 96th Congress, and at this writing there was every indication that it would,[53] then approval of *a* bill by the Senate this year would be very helpful in the next Congress. For this reason it is highly probable that the administration and its supporters were willing to accept any compromise, no matter how detrimental technically it might have been to the thrust of the original proposal, if that meant the administration could achieve a victory on hospital cost containment. It is also highly likely that the victory was due in part to the administration's willingness to compromise, and to the view of individual senators that the bill was not going anywhere at that time.

The problem with this approach is that it tends to ignore whatever basic problems exist with the cost containment methodology included in the bill, and this fact does not suggest that improvements in the bill will be forthcoming in the 96th Congress. Whatever underlying difficulties may exist with the bill are hidden under either a barrage of rhetoric terming hospitals "obese," or are lost to view because legitimate concerns are dealt with through special exemptions or weakening amendments like legislative vetoes. The next chapter discusses some of those concerns as they relate to the basic mandatory cost containment proposals.

IV | Assessment

11 | Conclusion

Evidence of the need for containing hospital costs, and the case for the Hospital Cost Containment bill, were summarized by Vice President Walter Mondale in a speech to a Conference on Health Care Costs:

> There are no villains in the story of rising health care costs. Instead it is a classic example of the famous Pogo cartoon, in which the character announces, "We have met the enemy and it is us." As . . . pointed out, our present health care system has no incentive to cut costs. It rewards spending and penalizes efficiency. Our hospitals compete for doctors and patients, not by offering lower prices but by offering more expensive equipment, new hospital wings, and every conceivable hospital service.
>
> Such a system encourages over-building. We have 100,000 empty hospital beds in this country, which cost $2 million a year to maintain. It encourages duplication of expensive equipment from hospital to hospital, which is underused. It encourages overhospitalization. One person in seven could be more cheaply treated at home in a less costly setting.
>
> No single individual is responsible for this waste and duplication, but all of us pay for the consequences. If we do not act to halt inflation in hospital costs, total spending for hospital care will balloon to $220 billion in less than ten years [from an estimated $66 billion in 1977], and the cost of a hospital stay will be more than $5,000 [as compared to an estimated $1400 in 1977]. Clearly, the time has come—indeed it has been here for a long time—to bite the bullet on hospital costs.[1]

Not surprisingly, the vice president termed the administration's proposed Hospital Cost Containment Act the "essential first step" in dealing with the problems of the health care system.

Notwithstanding the eloquence of the vice president, and the research evidence available to substantiate his points, the Congress was not able to take that "first step." The reasons are varied, and not always clear, but those which can be presented fall into three general categories: technical, political, and philosophical.

Technical Problems

Most of the technical problems with the bill were presented earlier. Steps were taken by one or more of the committees to ameliorate those problems. For example, the original bill (administration) implied a rate of increase less than the prevailing rate of inflation. Both the Rogers and Rostenkowski subcommittees removed that effect by changing the revenue limit to a flat 150 percent of the GNP deflator and by applying the limit on a compound basis, although these provisions would only apply if the Voluntary Effort fails in the Rostenkowski bill. Similarly, the exceptions process was broadened to deal with changes in the distribution of purchasers, and undesignated gifts were removed from the exceptions process.

Although these and other changes cut the estimated savings under the program by 41 percent,[2] thereby softening its provisions substantially, they do not deal with many of the most important technical problems of the administration's proposal. A significant problem in passing this legislation is that it applies relatively arbitrary controls in a nonspecific fashion to the production of an important, highly regarded set of personal services. There is no responsible way to defend, or attack, the use of the 150 percent of the GNP deflator limit, or the administration's original declining limit, because the necessary evidence was not made available, if it exists. Of course, it may not be possible to arrive at a limit for hospital costs which is actually based upon an acceptable measure of need and, therefore, it may be necessary to use an arbitrary figure and assess its impact after the fact. Regardless, in terms of the present controversy, the lack of any acceptable measure of the proper level of resources which should be provided for hospital care made it easy for opponents to attack the proposal, and difficult for proponents to defend it.

The difficulty faced by proponents can be demonstrated through an attempt to assess the impact of the hospital cost containment bill, based upon the available data. HEW now estimates that in the aggregate, the actual allowable increase in hospital revenue would have been 12.1 percent in fiscal year 1979 if the bill had passed in 1978. In comparison, AHA states that hospital costs went up 15.6 percent in 1977. The effect of cutting total costs by 3.5 percent was, therefore, the question at hand.

One possible effect is that hospitals would cut into their "profit" margins, as they did under the Economic Stabilization Program. There does appear to be some slack in this area since in 1976 the profit margin for all U.S. hospitals (defined as net total revenue over total expenses) amounted to 2.72 percent or $1.225 billion.[3] Theoretically, if all U.S.

hospitals could share their profits, and were willing just to break even, they would only have to cut another .78 percent of their total revenue to meet the limits. There are two problems with this proposition. Obviously, not all hospitals have the same margin of revenue over costs; the range by state is from a high of 10.22 percent for all Louisiana hospitals to a low of minus 1.16 percent in New York; and, of course, not all hospitals in Louisiana have that high a margin.[4] The uneven distribution of profit margins is further evidenced by a recent HEW study which found that many public hospitals, and some community hospitals, were forced to cut back services due to increased costs, a signal that their financial position was not strong.[5]

The second problem is that it is unreasonable to expect hospitals simply to break even, as most hospital administrators will want to insure that some profit margin is available to deal with unforeseen contingencies. For these reasons, a flat revenue cap will force some hospitals to take a hard look at the services they produce, as well as the intensity increases which occur each year in most hospitals, while others will be able to get by, at least in the short term, by spending down their margin from earlier years. The problem in assessing the ability of hospitals to "get by" in the short term is that data are available only in an aggregated form, and it is most difficult if not impossible to assess the impact on the financial position of an individual hospital. Furthermore, one needs to know why those hospitals in poor financial shape were having problems; it may be that they are the ones providing duplicative or unneeded services, or are producing services of poor quality and, therefore, are having trouble competing for physicians.

The lack of a reliable data base also makes it difficult to assess the impact of the bill's revenue limits on intensity increases. As noted above, there is some controversy over how much inflation exists in the costs hospitals face for providing the present level of services. AHA's measure of hospital input prices (Hospital Costs Index) shows prices rising at an annual rate of 10.6 percent since the end of the Economic Stabilization Program, although the 1977 rate of increase has slowed to 8.6 percent.[6] In contrast, the Consumer Price Index shows all prices rising at an annual rate of 7.5 percent since the Economic Stabilization Program, with hospital service charges rising at 12.9 percent and semiprivate room rates rising at 14.6 percent.[7] AHA claims that the CPI understates price changes in the goods hospitals must buy because of their unique market basket. It also claims that input price changes are overstated in the hospital service charge and semiprivate room rate indices because they do not differentiate between pure price increases and quality and intensity increases. However, AHA's indices also mask some quality and intensity increases, and the Hospital Costs Index overstates pure price inflation to some extent. It is possible, therefore, to conclude that pure price inflation in hospital costs is rising at a pace somewhere in between AHA's claimed rate of 8.6 percent and the CPI's present annual rate of 7.9 percent.

Nonetheless, if one accepts AHA's index, hospitals would be able to tolerate the proposed revenue limits if they eliminated all intensity increases. This point is established in the analysis conducted by Feldstein[8] in support of the National Council of Community Hospitals' proposal to freeze all increases in full-time equivalent employees. Although it was stated that a freeze on employment by itself was not likely to control costs, since administrators could shift increased expenditures elsewhere, the analysis concluded that if hospital administrators were willing to forego or defer all expenditures for new employees, the rate of increase in total hospital costs would be reduced to about the same rate proposed by the administration. Of course not every hospital has been hiring at the same rate in the past, so freezing new employment would not reduce the rate of cost increase in every hospital at the same rate. The evidence only suggests that some of the necessary cost reductions could be accomplished in this way.

An additional manner in which hospitals could contain costs would be to reduce the rate of increase in hospital beds, or eliminate or defer all capital expenditures. Assessing the impact of such reductions is difficult because again the available data are aggregated on too gross a level and, therefore, the impact on operating costs can only be estimated. The best that can be said is that the 1975–1977 average annual capital investment was \$5.2 billion.[9] Using HEW's rule of thumb that \$1.00 in capital expenditure produces \$.50 in annual operating expenses, this rate of capital investment translates into a \$2.6 billion increase in annual operating costs or about 4.3 percent of the projected 1978 base of \$60 billion in hospital expenditures. If hospitals eliminate or defer all capital investment, the rate of increase in total operating costs could be reduced to about 11.8 percent.

Two problems exist with this estimate. First, it is very much a "ballpark" estimate. Second, it is unlikely that all capital expenditures can be eliminated or deferred, as many hospitals presently are in violation of code standards, especially the newer regulations relating to access for the handicapped. A more likely possibility is that most construction for new beds could be halted considering that an estimated 100,000 excess beds presently exist. Of the total capital spending, \$1.2 billion is associated with new beds; if no new beds were constructed, operating cost increases would be reduced by about 1 percent. It is also important to note that $1.4 billion was spent on new equipment, some of which is duplicative and unneeded; some of that amount could be eliminated, but a problem is the difficulty in predicting the dollar amount to be saved.

Any reduction in capital expenditures most likely would result from application of the revenue cap rather than the capital expenditure limit, because the capital expenditure limit applies only to those expenditures which are reviewable by certificate of need agencies; this amounted to an average of $4.4 billion in the period from 1975 to 1977. Moreover, there are many approved expenditures already in the works and HEW estimates that it will take until 1981 to get total reviewable expenditures down to the proposed $2.5 billion limit.[10]

This is about as far as it is possible to venture in estimating the impact of the proposed revenue limitations in light of available data. As can be seen, the gross level at which the data are aggregated, and the insensitivity of the resulting estimates, make it very difficult to assert with any certainty what the impact of the administration's proposal would have been; this makes the proposal vulnerable to attack. Moreover, in consideration of the variation among hospitals, it is most difficult if not impossible to identify which hospitals will be able to take advantage of the possible areas of cost savings suggested by the data. It can be stated, as HEW has, only that rates of increase are similar for different hospitals even though the underlying cost structure on which the increases are based varies widely. Unfortunately, even this point is hard to accept since the data available indicate that small hospitals (4,000 admissions annually or less) have a rate of increase 1.2 percent higher than large hospitals.[11]

Nonetheless, there are some indications that hospitals could live within the revenue limitations without a serious impact upon health. First, four states which do not have mandatory control programs had a rate of increase less than 12 percent in 1977. Second, New York State has reduced per admission cost increases to only 2.8 percent in 1976, while reducing hospital net losses from $385 million to $60 million, and there have been no reports that this reduction caused a negative impact upon health status. Four other mandatory state programs also have been able to achieve a rate of increase less than 12 percent, although their results have not been as dramatic as New York's.[12] It is important to recognize, however, that except for New York's, these programs do not use a flat revenue cap, but treat hospitals individually. Similarly, the four states having a significant operating history in hospital cost control (New York,

Maryland, Connecticut, and Massachusetts) started with a very high base relative to other states and, therefore, could be said to have more "fat" which they could safely reduce or eliminate.

Another important consideration regarding a hospital's ability to tolerate the cap is the length of the program. The evidence indicates that, in general, input costs are rising less than the annual revenue limit which the program would impose. For this reason, the important concern is the length of time hospitals can defer needed increases in quality, intensity, and quantity of their services. In consideration of experience under the Economic Stabilization Program, it would seem possible for hospitals to defer some of their expenditures for a period of two to four years. Unfortunately, the administration's proposal was not particularly explicit about when a permanent program replacing the transitional revenue limitation would be ready, or what shape it would take.

It is important to note that the administration's original bill contained a provision stating that the secretary of HEW would submit to Congress by March 1, 1978 his recommendations for permanent reforms in health care financing and delivery; that date has passed. Now, instead of having completed the task set forth in the bill originally introduced, HEW's March 17, 1978 briefing document stated that it expected the permanent program "to be ready in two to three years."[13]

The administration, therefore, left its supporters in the Congress without the one crucial piece of evidence which could substantially remove the need for a more explicit assessment of the impact of the revenue limits and blunt the critics' attacks. After all, the Voluntary Effort proposed that hospitals bring the rate of increase down to 12 percent by 1979, and that is close to the rate being proposed for the mandatory program. If the hospital administrators think it can be done, one has to assume that it is possible. However, they too are thinking in terms of a temporary effort, since AHA's letter to hospital administrators asked, for example, for reductions or *postponement* of capital expenditures.[14]

The lack of a general proposal for a permanent program is the largest single technical obstruction to the passage of a cost containment bill. Nonetheless, the bill would still face serious problems even if all the technical problems could be solved and the specific data base existed to prove that the revenue and capital limits were justified and necessary in the long run.

Political Problems

Perhaps the most obvious political problem in passing a cost containment bill is that the debate is not often based upon consideration of objective data, but upon the political clout of the person presenting a viewpoint or upon the political philosophy of the particular congressman to whom the information is presented. An example of this is the issue of pass-throughs for labor or for other costs like food and energy proposed during the second Ways and Means subcommittee mark-up sessions. The AHA cost index, information contained in the Council on Wage and Price Stability report on wages, and the information on wages presented by the Maryland rate review commission, all strongly indicate that pass-throughs are unjustified and unnecessary.

The AHA index, with all its technical problems, suggests that *all* hospital input costs are inflating at a lower rate than the revenue limit, and the wage data indicate that the hospital workers are better paid than their counterparts in private industry. Moreover, in the case of wages, the percentage of total hospital costs attributable to wages has been steadily dropping. For these reasons, pass-throughs would be inflationary and contrary to the intent of a program designed to put constraints on resource use in hospitals. Nonetheless, the hospital lobbies pushed for nonlabor pass-throughs, and the result was to include them in one version of the cost containment bill. Similarly, labor lobbyists have pushed for the mandatory wage pass-through; again, it was included in one version. Thus, even the administration was willing to accept the mandatory wage pass-through so that labor would support the bill.

Philosophical Problems

These problems with passing the bill are difficult to evaluate but they certainly exist. There is something of a backlash against federal regulation occurring at this time, mostly as a result of the tremendous increase in the federal presence resulting from the actions of President Johnson and the Great Society legislative program. Many, including a number of congressmen, would like to reverse the trend towards greater federal regulation and larger federal involvement in the affairs of individual citizens, corporations, and state and local governments. The hospital cost containment proposal is seen by many as an example of the federal government's efforts to intrude into everyone's lives, notwithstanding the need for restraint in health care cost increases. Moreover, the provider lobbies have been able to inject into the debate their Voluntary Effort, which involves no extension of government power and, if it works, could restrain fiscal 1978 and fiscal 1979 costs at about the same level proposed by the mandatory program, as modified. The lobbyists have been effective in getting congressmen to understand that standby controls will interfere with private efforts and should be defeated. This is a very seductive argument especially if the listener is generally opposed to extensions of federal regulatory powers. Opponents can also point to existing federal health regulation activities (health planning, certificate of need, and the PSROs) and say that enough is enough; existing efforts should be left to do their jobs, and that will be sufficient.

Perhaps the major philosophical argument is the one alluded to in the chapter on previous governmental control efforts. This issue is that health is a personal, localized service, and decisions concerning the use of resources should be left to local people, although this argument may really reflect general opposition to resource constraints on health care rather than a questioning of the proper locus for decision making. It is also a very persuasive argument since most members of the House of Representatives are local politicians whose viewpoints necessarily have geographical restrictions. This does not constitute a criticism, as they are elected to represent the people of their district, and, on issues about which they truly care, most congressmen are capable of rising above purely local interests. But just as the third party payment system protects consumers and providers from the consequences of their poor economic decisions in regard to health care, it also removes any local incentive to deal with rising costs. Therefore, except for the congressmen who are expecially interested in health, there is very little incentive to support an unpalatable measure like cost containment; it is an issue from which few votes will be gained.

It is also interesting to note that political philosophy may inhibit an attempt to understand and correctly interpret the provisions of the cost containment proposal. An example of this recently appeared in *Congress Today*, the official magazine of the National Republican Congressional Committee.[15] In an article entitled "Hospital Hoodwink," which attacked the bill's increased federal regulation, it was stated that hospitals would be forced to cut back their revenues and that mandatory controls would be imposed if they did "not make the required two percent cut." The point is that no *cut* in revenues is proposed at all; rather, hospitals are required to cut the *rate of increase* by 2 percent under the Rostenkowski proposal to which the article was alluding.

Future Outlook

A combination of strong opposition, weak public support, and a lack of credible information led to the demise of the Hospital Cost Containment Act in 1978. Instead, the country is left with a Voluntary Effort controlled by those who must accept most of the responsibility for increasing hospital expenditures in the first place. Moreover, the stimulus which reasonably can be concluded to have initiated the voluntary program, the threat of federal controls, has been removed. The question then is, can the Voluntary Effort continue its early success?

HEW Secretary Joseph Califano termed the voluntary program "a false promise to the American people," and noted that although hospitals have had ample opportunity to restrain increases voluntarily, "the evidence shows they have not been effective."[16] The problem for the Voluntary Effort and its three national sponsors (the American Medical Association, the American Hospital Association, and the Federation of American Hospitals) is that they find themselves in a position analogous to that of the president when he attempts to "jawbone" price increases or decrease union wage demands. These three sponsoring organizations must persuade several thousand individual actors in the hospital field to slow the rate of increase in their costs in order to protect the collective good, i.e., to avoid the imposition of federal or state controls. The problem in persuading a group is that any benefits of the collective action will accrue to all members regardless of their contribution. So although the hospitals and the physicians may have a strong desire as a group to insure the success of the Voluntary Effort, the removal of the threat which would have affected every member may mean that individuals may begin to ignore the effort's goals. To the extent that enough members of the group decide that their individual financial situation is unique, or decide that their actions will have little or no impact upon the group average, it can be surmised that prices will tend to rise and the Voluntary Effort will fail.[17]

Nevertheless, in view of the problem which the providers themselves are attempting to solve, it is important that the providers are at least recognizing their responsibility to act. It is possible that their recognition of the problem may serve in some respects to facilitate the debate over restraints on health costs. It is certainly true that the deliberations and debate thus far have raised more questions than have been answered about how the health care system should be structured, and thus any assistance from health care providers will undoubtedly be most welcome.

It is also true that for the moment Congress has decided that the only available option is to monitor the Voluntary Effort, thus leaving the question of why that particular decision was reached at this time. Did Congress merely bow to the power of the special interests, or were there compelling and legitimate reasons for rejecting the administration's proposal? The answer is necessarily based upon opinion, but there are clearly many political, technical, and philosophical problems which obstructed the passage of the bill. Certainly provider lobbyists applied a great deal of pressure to the Congress on this issue, but their efforts were immeasurably aided by the fact that the third party payment system immunizes the public from the impact of inflation in health care expenditures, thus removing the crucial counter pressure which might have caused Congress to act differently. More importantly, the provider lobbies represent an industry whose product is thought to be a basic right of every citizen. For this reason, the burden of providing proof beyond the reasonable doubts of congressmen was not on the hospitals and the physicians; it was on those who proposed to curtail the portion of the nation's resources going to health.

One serious problem in developing the case for hospital cost containment is that the data base upon which the decisions are being made is abysmal. It may be that the Social Security Administration or HEW's Office of the Actuary has data on the impact of a 12 percent revenue limit, but it has not been forthcoming to Congress. For example, there is little evidence available on the number of underutilized specialized hospital units, or on their distribution, or on their cost. It certainly seems possible that HEW could use its own National Health Planning Guidelines to identify just how many excess beds and units exist in the categories on which guidelines have been written, and join that information with the cost data collected by HEW to arrive at a fairly specific estimate of the costs of excess capacity. Similarly, the Commerce Department's construction cost index could be used in conjunction with the planning guidelines to arrive at the costs of needed capital expenditures for those categories. Furthermore, cost data could be used to arrive at an estimate of the operating cost impact of those needed expenditures. Without uniform reporting, if not uniform accounting, hospital costs are not strictly comparable; moreover, the guidelines do not cover every category of capital expenditure, so the results of this analysis would necessarily be an estimate. These estimates, however, would be far preferable to the crude estimates stated earlier in this chapter.

This lack of information with the resultant impairment of the cost containment debate further serves to underline the importance of the regional health planning system, the PSROs, and the federally supported cooperative health statistics centers. The Health Systems Plans and the Annual Implementation Plans produced by health planners which are just now starting to become available should provide an important first step towards improving the ability to assess the need for capital improvements, and to identify the amount of excess capacity at the national level. Similarly, the Profile Analyses which the PSROs are supposed to be producing would provide an important tool for identifying unnecessary and inapproppriate utilization. Aggregating these data within the cooperative statistics centers and improving the distribution of this information would undoubtedly prove to be of great assistance in selectively identifying what could and could not safely be eliminated from the system.

It is also true that much more could be done to institute the kinds of linkage mechanisms among health planning, utilization review, and state rate review where it exists to exploit to the fullest extent the data-collection mechanisms possible under these programs. These efforts to improve the understanding of the health care system are essential if a cost containment system is to do what it is supposed to do.

Another conclusion is that it is necessary to move as aggressively as possible toward the development of a permanent control system. The large concern about the need to avoid a negative impact on needed health care can only be answered through the design of a more specific and more sophisticated approach than that contained in the Hospital Cost Containment Act. Moreover, in consideration of the difficulty in defining the need of the population for more health care services, particularly secondary and tertiary services, and the difficulty in defining the size of the share of national resources which should be allocated to health, it is clear that the only way in which the nation can make these important decisions is through a long process of debate. The debate must be based upon reasonably good information, and conducted in a responsible fashion.

It must also be recognized that although the Hospital Cost Containment Act did not pass during the 95th Congress, it already has had a definite impact upon the health care delivery system; one example is the proposal of the Voluntary Effort. In consideration of past provider actions, it is hard to believe that the Voluntary Effort would have been implemented if the president had not proposed the Hospital Cost Containment Act. Another important example is a recent announcement made by AMA Executive Vice President James Sammons: "The AMA House of Delegates has endorsed the development of educational programs designed to increase the understanding and awareness of medical school faculty, medical students, and the housestaff of the cost of health and medical care. The House has also supported options for increasing the cost awareness of physicians in practice."[18]

Moreover, the president's proposal has raised the stakes on efforts to control health care costs. A few months ago, the AMA was fighting hard against the national health planning act. Now that initiative seems relatively benign next to the hospital cost containment proposal, and physicians and hospitals are pointing to the planning act as a reason why a cost containment bill is unnecessary.

Finally, the president's proposal has finally begun the national debate which was so clearly needed on the level of resources provided to health. The Hospital Cost Containment Act may not have done as much as hoped to change the underlying structure of the system. It did not even pass but, nonetheless, it demonstrates that there is recognition of the need to reallocate health care resources. It is an unusual phenomenon for an American president, especially a Democratic one, to propose that the nation tighten its collective belt and lower its expectations for social services. The president has proposed that it be done; therefore, the issue finally is being faced by all of the participants in the health care delivery system. It is true that there is still a large educational program which must be conducted among the public and its representatives in local, state, and federal governments. It also is necessary to commit a far larger effort to the design of a more workable and more equitable program than that proposed through the Hospital Cost Containment Act. Nevertheless, the health care cost problem will not go away by itself, and it can be asserted that, once started, the job will work its way to completion. It must be sooner rather than later so that funds which are being consumed by inefficiency, duplication, and unnecessary care can be applied to some of the truly important health care service problems of the country.

Appendix

Appendix
Guide to the Bills

Bill Number and Sponsor	Comments
H.R. 6575 (Rogers) S. 1391 (Kennedy)*	The original Administration bill (H.R. 6575/S.1391) never received final approval by two of the four committees to which it was referred; therefore, it died in committee.
H.R. 8121 (Rogers)	No final action was taken on this bill as it was introduced to publicize its proposed amendments to H.R. 6575; there was no identical bill in the Senate.
H.R.8337 (Rostenkowski)	No final action was taken on this bill as it was introduced to publicize its proposed amendments to H.R. 6575; there was no identical bill in the Senate.
S. 1878 (Schweiker)	This was the first state-oriented bill, some of its provisions were included in the Human Resources Committee version of S. 1391; there was no identical bill in the House of Representatives.
H.R. 8687 (Carter)	A bill similar to S. 1878, some of its provisions were included in the Subcommittee on Health and the Environment version of H.R. 6575; there was no identical bill in the Senate.
H.R. 7079 (Rogers) S. 1470 (Talmadge)*	The original Talmadge bill was introduced as a courtesy by Rogers in the House of Representatives; the Finance Committee added a revised version of this bill to H.R. 5285 which passed the Senate on October 12, 1978.
S. 1391 (as reported by the Committee on Human Resources)	Title I of this bill was defeated by the Senate as an amendment to H.R. 5285 on October 12, 1978.

---

*Identical bill.

H.R. 9717 (Rogers)	This bill is the version of H.R. 6575 actually considered by the Committee on Interstate and Foreign Commerce, as reported to the Committee by the Subcommittee on Health and the Environment.
Broyhill Amendment	This was the most significant amendment approved by the Committee on Interstate and Foreign Commerce in reporting H.R. 6575 to the House of Representatives. However, the amended version of H.R. 6575 was never considered by the House of Representatives due to the lack of action by its Committee on Ways and Means.
H.R. 5285 (as reported by the Senate Finance Committee)	This bill was stripped of its original purpose by the Finance Committee, amended with a revised text of S. 1470, and passed by the Senate on October 12, 1978.
Nelson Amendment	This amendment was approved by the Senate during consideration of H.R. 5285 on October 12, 1978; the amendment provided for mandatory controls if voluntary efforts failed.

References

Chapter 1

1. Jonathan Spivak, "Where Do We Go From Here?" in *Conference on National Health Insurance, University of Pennsylvania, 1970*, ed. Robert D. Eilers and Sue S. Moyerman (Homewood, IL: R. D. Irwin for the Leonard Davis Institute of Health Economics, University of Pennsylvania, 1971), p. 272.
2. R.M. Gibson and C.R. Fisher, "National Health Expenditures, Fiscal Year 1977," *Social Security Bulletin* 41 (July 1978): 3-20.
3. U.S. Congress, Senate, *National Health Planning and Development and Health Facilities Assistance Act of 1974*, S. Rept. 93-1285 to Accompany S. 2994, 93rd Cong., 2d sess., 1974.
4. Victor R. Fuchs, "Health Care and the U.S. Economic System: An Essay in Abnormal Psychology," in *Economic Aspects of Health Care*, ed. J.B. McKinlay (New York: Prodist for the Milbank Memorial Fund, 1973), pp. 95-122.
5. Victor M. Zink, "Greater Effort Needed to Control Costs," *Hospitals* 50 (March 16, 1976): 65-67.
6. Council on Wage and Price Stability, *The Complex Puzzle of Rising Health Care Costs: Can the Private Sector Fit It Together?* (Washington, D.C.: Executive Office of the President, December 1976), pp. 2-3.
7. Uwe Reinhardt, "Proposed Changes in the Organization of Health Care Delivery: An Overview and Critique," *Milbank Memorial Fund Quarterly* 51 (Spring 1973): 169-222.
8. Victor R. Fuchs, *Who Shall Live?* (New York: Basic Books, 1974), pp. 52-54.
9. Ibid., p. 53.
10. R. Auster, I. Leveson, and D. Sarachek, "The Production of Health, an Exploratory Study," *Journal of Human Resources* 4 (Fall 1969): 441-436.
11. R. Logan et al., "Dynamics of Medical Care: The Liverpool Study into Use of Hospital Resources," (Memoir No. 14, London School of Hygiene, 1972) cited by Walter McClure, *Reducing Excess Hospital Capacity* (Excelsior, Minnesota: Interstudy, 1976), p. 9.
12. John Wennberg and Alan Gittelsohn, "Small Area Variations in Health Care Delivery," *Science* 182 (December 1973): 1102-1108.
13. Walsh McDermott, Kurt W. Deuschle, and Clifford R. Barnett, "Health Care Experiment at Many Farms," *Science* 175 (January 7, 1972): 23-31.
14. Lee Benham and Alexandra Benham, "The Impact of Incremental Medical Services on Health Status 1963-1970," in *Equity in Health Services*, ed. Ronald Anderson et al. (Cambridge, Massachusetts: Ballinger, 1975).

15. K. Astvad et al., "Mortality from Acute Myocardial Infarction Before and After Establishment of a Coronary Care Unit," *British Medical Journal*, March 23, 1974, pp. 567–569.
16. Fuchs, "Health Care and the U.S. Economic System," p. 98.
17. Karen Davis, *Health and the War on Poverty: A Ten Year Appraisal* (Washington, D.C.: Brookings Institution, 1977).
18. Congressional Budget Office, *Expenditures for Health Care: Federal Programs and their Effects* (Washington, D.C.: U.S. Government Printing Office, 1977), p. ix.
19. McClure, *Hospital Capacity*, p. 1.
20. U.S. Department of Health, Education, and Welfare, Public Health Service, Health Resources Administration, *Health: United States 1976–1977* (Washington, D.C.: U.S. Government Printing Office, 1977), p. vi.
21. U.S. Congress, House, Committee on Ways and Means, Subcommittee on Health and Committee on Interstate and Foreign Commerce, Subcommittee on Health and the Environment, *President's Hospital Cost Containment Proposal, Joint Hearings on H.R. 6575*, 95th Cong., 1st sess., 1977, p. 14.
22. Ibid.
23. Joseph Newhouse, *Income and Medical Care Expenditures Across Countries: Is Medical Care at the Margin a Luxury Good?* (Santa Monica: The Rand Corporation, 1976).
24. Reinhardt, "On the Other Hand," *Medical World News*, February 21, 1977, p. 108.
25. "Hospitals Headlines," *Hospitals* 57 (February 16, 1977): 17–18.

Chapter 2

1. R.M. Gibson and C.R. Fisher, "National Health Expenditures, Fiscal Year 1977," *Social Security Bulletin* 41 (July 1978): 3–20.
2. American Hospital Association, *Hospital Statistics*, 1978 ed. (Chicago: American Hospital Association, 1978).
3. Idem, *Hospital Statistics*, various editions, 1951–1978.
4. Ibid.

Chapter 3

1. American Hospital Association, *Hospital Statistics*, 1977 ed. (Chicago: American Hospital Association, 1977), p. xiii.
2. Martin S. Feldstein, *The Rising Cost of Hospital Care* (Washington, D.C.: Information Resources, Press, 1971), pp. 16–17.
3. Karen Davis and Richard W. Foster, *Community Hospitals: Inflation in the Pre-Medicare Period*, Social Security Administration, Office of Research and Statistics Research Report No. 41 (Washington, D.C.: U.S. Government Printing Office, 1972).
4. S. Lee, "Teaching Hospitals: Alone or Together," *Bulletin of the New York Academy of Medicine* 48 (December 1972): 1267–1473.

5. R.D. Elkin, "Recognition and Negotiation Under Taft-Hartley," *Hospital Progress* 55 (December 1974): 50–53, 63.

6. C.S. Bunker, "A Study to Determine the Impact of Unionization and the Threat Thereof on New York City's Voluntary Nonprofit Hospitals" (Ph.D. dissertation, George Washington University, 1968), pp. 94–99.

7. Stuart Altman and Joseph Eichenholz, "Inflation in the Health Industry—Causes and Cures," in *Health: A Victim or Cause of Inflation?* ed. Michael Zubkoff (New York: Prodist for the Milbank Memorial Fund, 1976), p.19.

8. Feldstein, *Rising Cost*, Chapter 5.

9. U.S. Congress, Senate, Committee on Human Resources, Subcommittee on Health and Scientific Research, *Hospital Cost Containment Act of 1977, Hearings on S. 1391*, 95th Cong., 1st sess., 1977, pp. 606–608.

10. Feldstein, *Rising Cost*, Chapter 5.

11. Karen Davis, "The Role of Technology, Demand, and Labor Markets in the Determination of Health Care Costs," in *The Economics of Health and Medical Care*, ed. Mark Perlman (New York: John Wiley and Sons, 1974), pp. 283–301 and idem, "Hospital Costs and the Medicare Program," *Social Security Bulletin* 36 (August 1973): 33.

12. Carol M. McCarthy, "Supply and Demand and Hospital Cost Inflation," *Medical Care Review* 33 (August 1976): 928.

13. Altman and Eichenholz, "Inflation in the Health Industry," p. 19.

14. Davis, "The Medicare Program," p. 35.

15. Idem, "Rising Hospital Costs: Possible Causes and Cures," *Bulletin of the New York Academy of Medicine* 48 (December 1972): 1361.

16. J. Krizay and A. Wilson, *The Patient as Consumer* (Lexington: Lexington Books, 1974), p. 103.

17. H.D. Lytton, "Recent Trends in the Federal Government: An Exploratory Study," *Review of Economics and Statistics* 41 (November 1959): 341–359.

18. Herbert E. Klarman, "Reimbursing the Hospital—The Difference the Third Party Makes," *Journal of Risk and Insurance* 36 (December 1969): 562.

19. Feldstein, *Rising Cost*, pp. 16–19.

20. R.A. Elnicki, "Effects of Phase II Price Controls on Hospital Services," *Health Services Research* 7 (Summer 1974): 106–117.

21. J. Cromwell, "Hospital Productivity Trends in Short-Term General Non-Teaching Hospitals," *Inquiry* 11 (September 1974): 181–187.

22. J.R. Jeffers and C.D. Siebert, "Measurement of Hospital Cost Variation: Case Mix, Service Intensity, and Input Productivity Factors," *Health Services Research* 9 (Winter 1974): 293–307.

23. R.A. Elnicki, "Hospital Productivity, Service Intensity, and Costs," *Health Services Research* 9 (Winter 1974): 289.

24. Davis, "Rising Hospital Costs," p. 1361.

25. John Alexander McMahon and David F. Drake, "Inflation and the Hospital," in *Health: A Victim or Cause of Inflation?* ed. Michael Zubkoff (New York: Prodist for the Milbank Memorial Fund, 1976), p. 136.

26. American Hospital Association, *Guide to the American Hospital Association's Program for Monitoring the Hospital Economy* (Chicago: American Hospital Association, Bureau of Research Services, 1974).

27. U.S. Congress, Senate, *Hearings on S. 1391,* p. 183.

28. P. Joseph Philip, James R. Jeffers, and Abdul Hai, "Indexes of Factor Input Price, Service Intensity, and Productivity for the Hospital Industry," in *"The Nature of Hospital Costs: Three Studies"* (Chicago: Hospital Research and Educational Trust, 1976) (processed). See also: P. Joseph Phillip, "Indices of Price and Intensity for the Hospital Industry," (Chicago: Hospital Research and Educational Trust, 1976) (processed); idem, "HCI-HII," *Hospital Financial Management,* April 1977, pp. 20–26; idem, "New AHA Indexes Provide Fairer View of Rising Costs," *Hospitals* 51 (July 16, 1977): 175–182.

29. Idem, "Indices of Price and Intensity," p. 6.

30. John Banes, Personal Communication, May 25, 1976.

31. See McCarthy, "Supply and Demand," p. 929.

32. Walter McClure, "The Medical System under National Health Insurance: Four Models," *Journal of Health Politics, Policy, and Law,* Spring 1976, p.32.

33. American Hospital Association, Hospital Statistics, 1977, ed., p. 4.

34. Ann Scitovsky and Nelda McCall, "Changes in the Costs of Treatment of Selected Illnesses," *Research Digest Series* (Washington, D.C.: Department of Health, Education, and Welfare, Public Health Service, Health Resources Administration, National Center for Health Services Research, 1976), pp. 14–17.

35. Herbert E. Klarman, "The Increased Cost of Hospital Care," in *The Economics of Health and Medical Care,* ed. S.J. Mushkin (Ann Arbor, Michigan: University of Michigan School of Public Health, Bureau of Public Health Economics, 1964), p. 247.

36. Davis and Foster, "Community Hospitals," p. 79 and Davis, "The Medicare Program," p. 23.

37. McCarthy, "Supply and Demand," p. 931.

38. U.S. Department of Health, Education, and Welfare, Public Health Service, Health Resources Administration, National Center for Health Statistics, *Health in the United States: A Chartbook, 1975,* (Washington, D.C.: U.S. Government Printing Office, 1975), p. 5.

39. Congressional Budget Office, *Expenditures for Health Care: Federal Programs and their Effects* (Washington, D.C.: U.S. Government Printing Office, 1977) p. ix.

40. Davis, "The Role of Technology."

41. John D. Thompson, Robert Fetter, and Charles Mross, "Case Mix and Resource Use," *Inquiry* 12 (December 1975): 300–312.

42. Scitovsky and McCall, *Changes in the Cost of Treatment.*

43. McClure, "The Medical Care System," p. 24.

44. Congressional Budget Office, *Expenditures for Health Care,* p. 25.

45. Council on Wage and Price Stability, *The Complex Puzzle of Rising Health Care Costs,* p. 9.

46. As reported in Joseph P. Newhouse, "Toward a Theory of Nonprofit Institutions: An Economic Model of a Hospital," *American Economic Review* 60 (March 1970): 70.

47. H. Goldstein, "Health and Medicine," in *The Economist Looks at Society*, ed. G. Schuckster and E. Dale, Jr. (Lexington: Xerox Publishing Co., 1973), p. 169.

48. Scitovsky and McCall, *Changes in the Cost of Treatment*, pp. 20–22.

49. C. Aring, "The Place of the Physician in Modern Society," *Journal of the American Medical Association* 228 (April 8, 1974): 177.

50. J. Maloney, "A Report on the Role of Economic Motivation in the Performance of Medical School Faculty," *Surgery* 68 (July 1970): 1.

51. McClure, "The Medical Care System," p. 33.

52. Paul Elwood quoted in Fuchs, *Who Shall Live?* (New York: Basic Books, 1974), p. 58.

53. J. Rapoport, "Diffusion of Technological Innovation in Hospitals: A Case Study of Nuclear Medicine," *Final Report*, Grant No. HS 01238 (Washington, D.C.: U.S. Department of Health, Education, and Welfare, Public Health Service, Health Resources Administration, National Center for Health Services Research, September 1976).

54. Mark V. Pauly and Michael A. Redisch, "The Not-for-Profit Hospital as a Physicians' Cooperative," *American Economic Review* 63 (March 1973): 87–100.

55. G. Drakos, "The Not-for-Profit Hospital as a Physicians' Cooperative: A Comment" (Université de Sherbrooke, 1973) (unpublished) cited in Phillip Jacobs, "A Survey of Economic Models of Hospitals," *Inquiry* 11 (June 1974): 97.

56. J. Buchanan and C. Lindsay, "Financing of Medical Care in the United States," in *Health Services Financing* (London: British Medical Association, 1970).

57. Ibid., p. 549.

58. Davis, "Rising Hospital Costs," p. 1364.

59. U.S. Department of Health, Education, and Welfare, "Justification of the $2.5 Billion Capital Expenditure Ceiling," Briefing Document provided to the Committee on Interstate and Foreign Commerce, Subcommittee on Health and the Environment during consideration of H.R. 6575, August 1977 (processed).

60. Judith R. Lave and Lester B. Lave, *The Hospital Construction Act: An Evaluation of the Hill-Burton Program, 1948–1973* (Washington, D.C.: American Enterprise Institute for Public Policy Research, May 1974).

61. American Hospital Association, *Hospital Statistics*, 1977 ed.

62. R.S. Kelling and P.C. Williams, "The Projected Response of the Capital Markets to Health Facilities Expenditures for the Years 1976–1981," paper presented at the Conference on Capital Formation for Health Facilities, University of Pittsburgh, Pittsburgh, Pennsylvania, November 1976 cited in Congressional Budget Office, *Expenditures for Health Care*, p. 20.

63. American Hospital Association, *Hospital Statistics*, 1977 ed.

64. Institute of Medicine, *Controlling the Supply of Hospital Beds, A Policy*

Statement (Washington, D.C.: National Academy of Sciences, October 1976).

65. See R. Schulz and J. Rose, "Can Hospitals Be Expected to Control Costs," *Inquiry* 10 (June 1973): 3.

66. R. Logan et al., "Dynamics of Medical Care: The Liverpool Study into Use of Hospital Resources," (Memoir No. 14, London School of Hygiene, 1972) cited by Walter McClure, *Reducing Excess Hospital Capacity* (Excelsior, Minnesota Interstudy, 1976), p. 57.

67. Herbert E. Klarman, "What Kind of Health Insurance Should the United States Choose," in *The U.S. Medical Care Industry: An Economists Point of View*, ed. J.D. Morreale (Ann Arbor, Michigan: University of Michigan, Graduate School of Business, Division of Research, 1974), p. 74.

68. Karen Davis, "Theories of Hospital Inflation: Some Empirical Evidence," *Journal of Human Resources* 8 (Spring 1973): 181–201.

69. Mark V. Pauly and David F. Drake, "Effect of Third-Party Methods of Reimbursement on Hospital Performance," in *Empirical Studies in Health Economics*, ed. Herbert E. Klarman (Baltimore: Johns Hopkins Press, 1970), pp. 297–314.

70. Fred J. Hellinger, "Hospital Charges and Medicare Reimbursement," *Inquiry* 12 (December 1975): 313–319.

71. Davis, "The Medicare Program," p. 35.

72. J. Simanis, "International Health Expenditures," *Social Security Bulletin* 33 (December 1970): 18.

73. Health Insurance Institute, *Source Book of Health Insurance Data 1977–1978* (Washington, D.C.: Health Insurance Institute, 1978).

74. Stephen G. Sudovar, Jr. and Kathleen Sullivan, *National Health Insurance Issues, the Unprotected Population* (New York: Ben Kubasik Inc. for Roche Laboratories, 1978), p. 2.

75. Ibid.

76. Marian Gornick, "Ten Years of Medicare: Impact on the Covered Population," *Social Security Bulletin* 39 (July 1976): 5.

77. Health Insurance Institute, *Source Book*.

78. Davis, "Rising Hospital Costs," p. 1355.

79. Martin Feldstein, "Hospital Cost Inflation: A Study of Nonprofit Price Dynamics," *American Economic Review* 61 (December 1971): 853–872.

80. David S. Salkever, "A Microeconomic Study of Hospital Cost Inflation," *Journal of Political Economy* 80 (November–December 1972): 1144–1166.

81. Davis, "The Medicare Program," p. 31.

82. Idem, "The Role of Technology," p. 285.

83. Idem, "Community Hospital Expenses and Revenues: Pre-Medicare Inflation," *Social Security Bulletin* 35 (October 1972): 3–19.

84. B.A. Weisbrod and R.J. Fiesler, "Hospitalization Insurance and Hospital Utilization," *American Economic Review* 51 (March 1961): 126–132.

85. Paul J. Felstein and Ruth M. Severson, "The Demand for Medical Care," in *Report of the Commission on the Cost of Medical Care*, Vol. 1 (Chicago: American Medical Association, 1964).

86. Paul J. Feldstein and W. John Carr, "The Effect of Income on Medical Care Spending," in *Proceedings of the Statistical Section*, American Statistical Association (1964).

87. Gerald D. Rosenthal, *The Demand for General Hospital Facilities* (Chicago: American Hospital Association, 1974).

88. Odin W. Anderson and J.J. Feldman, *Family Medical Costs and Voluntary Health Insurance: A Nationwide Survey* (New York: Blakiston, 1956).

89. Ronald Andersen and Lee Benham, "Factors Affecting the Relationship Between Family Income and Medical Care Consumption," in *Empirical Studies in Health Economics*, ed. Herbert E. Klarman (Baltimore: Johns Hopkins Press, 1970), pp. 73–95.

90. Joseph P. Newhouse and Charles E. Phelps, "Price and Income Elasticity for Medical Care Services," in *The Economics of Health and Medical Care*, ed. Mark Perlman (New York: John Wiley and Sons, 1974), pp. 139–161.

91. Bernard Friedman, "A Test of Alternative Demand-Shift Responses to the Medicare Program," in *The Economics of Health and Medical Care*, ed. Mark Perlman (New York: John Wiley and Sons, 1974), pp. 234–247.

92. Scitovsky and McCall, *Changes in the Cost of Treatment*, p. 18.

93. Hyman Joseph, "Hospital Insurance and Moral Hazard," *Journal of Human Resources* 7 (Spring 1972): 152–161.

94. Gerald D. Rosenthal, "Price Elasticity of Demand for Short-Term General Hospital Services," in *Empirical Studies in Health Economics*, ed. Herbert E. Klarman (Baltimore: Johns Hopkins Press, 1970), pp. 101–117.

95. McClure, "The Medical Care System," p. 36.

96. U.S. Department of Health, Education, and Welfare, Public Health Service, Health Resources Administration, National Center for Health Statistics, *Health, United States—1976-1977 Chartbook* (Washington, D.C.: U.S. Government Printing Office, 1977), p. 24.

97. Gornick, "Ten Years of Medicare," p. 10.

98. John Wennberg, "PSRO and the Relationship Among Health Need, Elective Surgery, and Health Status," *Perspectives in Health Policy* 2 (August 1975): 8

99. Charles Lewis, "Variations in the Incidence of Surgery," *New England Journal of Medicine* 281 (October 16, 1969): 880.

100. Avedis V. Donabedian, "An Evaluation of Prepaid Group Practice," *Inquiry* 6 (September 1969): 3; M. Corbin and A. Krute, "Some Aspects of Medicare Experiences with Group Practice Prepayment Plans," *Social Security Bulletin* 36 (March 1973): 3; Milton Roemer and William Shonick, "HMO Performance: The Recent Evidence," *Milbank Memorial Fund Quarterly* 51 (Summer 1973): 271; and Robert Brook, "Critical Issues in the Assessment of Quality of Care," *Journal of Medical Education* 48, part 2 (April 1973): 114.

101. Milton Roemer and Max Shain, *Hospital Utilization Under Insurance* (Chicago: American Hospital Association, 1950).

102. J. Joel May, "Utilization of Health Services and the Availability of Resources," in *Equity in Health Services*, ed. Ronald Andersen et al.

(Cambridge, Massachusetts: Ballinger, 1975).

103. M. Feldstein, "Hospital Cost Inflation."

104. Rita Nickerson et al., "Doctors Who Perform Operations," *New England Journal of Medicine* 295 (October 21 and October 28, 1976): 921–926, 982–989.

105. Walter W. Hauck et al., "Surgeons in the United States," *Journal of the American Medical Association* 236 (October 1976): 1964–1971.

106. Victor R. Fuchs and Marcia J. Kramer, *Determinants of Expenditures for Physicians' Services in the United States, 1948–1968* (New York: National Bureau of Economic Research, 1972).

107. R.G. Evans, "Supplier Induced Demand: Some Empirical Evidence and Implications," paper prepared for the International Economic Association, Tokyo Conference on Economics of Health and Medical Care, April 1973, cited by Lave, Lave, and Leinhardt, "Medical Manpower Models: Need, Demand, and Supply," *Inquiry* 12 (June 1975): 97–125.

Chapter 4

1. Paul B. Ginsburg, "Inflation and Economic Stabilization Program," in *Health: A Victim or Cause of Inflation?* ed. Michael Zubkoff (New York: Prodist for the Milbank Memorial Fund, 1976), p. 35.

2. U.S. Government, Federal Register, *Code of Federal Regulations*, sec. 300.18, Preamble to Title 6, *Federal Register* 36 (December 31, 1971), pp. 25384–25385.

3. Idem, *Code of Federal Regulations*, sec. 300.18, *Federal Register* 37 (September 13, 1972), pp. 18548–18549.

4. Idem, *Code of Federal Regulations*, sec. 300.18, *Federal Register* 37 (July 1972), pp. 14312–14313.

5. Ginsburg, "The Economic Stabilization Program," p. 46.

6. Paul J. Feldstein, *An Empirical Investigation of the Marginal Costs of Hospital Services* (Chicago: University of Chicago Press, 1961).

7. Judith R. Lave and Lester B. Lave, "Hospital Cost Functions," *American Economic Review* 60 (June 1970): 379–395. See also Joseph Lipscomb, Ira E. Raskin, and Joseph Eichenholz, "The Use of Marginal Cost Estimates in Hospital Cost Containment Policy," in *Hospital Cost Containment: Selected Notes for Future Policy*, ed. Michael Zubkoff, Ira E. Raskin, and Ruth S. Hanft (New York: Prodist for the Milbank Memorial Fund, 1978), pp. 514–537.

8. Congressional Budget Office, *Expenditures for Health Care: Federal Programs and their Effects* (Washington, D.C.: U.S. Government Printing Office, 1977), p. 42.

9. Ginsburg, "The Economic Stabilization Program," p. 47.

10. Ibid., p. 50.

11. Stuart Altman; Joseph Eichenholz, "Inflation in the Health Industry—Causes and Cures," in *Health: A Victim or Cause of Inflation?* ed. Michael Zubkoff (New York: Prodist for the Milbank Memorial Fund, 1976), p. 22.

12. American Hospital Association, *Hospital Statistics*, 1977 ed.

13. Altman and Eichenholz, "Inflation in the Health Industry," pp. 23–25.

14. Ibid., pp. 26–27.

15. U.S. Department of Health, Education, and Welfare, Health Care Financing Administration, *Abstracts of State Legislated Hospital Cost Containment Programs* (Washington, D.C.: Health Care Financing Administration, May 1978).

16. U.S. Congress, House, *Voluntary Hospital Cost Containment Act of 1978*, H. Rept. 95–1789, Part I to Accompany H.R. 6575, 95th Cong., 2d sess., 1978, p. 33.

17. U.S. Congress, House, Committee on Interstate and Foreign Commerce, *Hospital Cost Containment*, Comm. Print 95–22, 95th Cong., 1st sess., 1977, p. 7.

18. John D. Thompson, Robert Fetter, and Charles Mross, "Case Mix and Resource Use," *Inquiry* 12 (December 1975): 300-312.

19. David S. Abernethy et al., *Prospective Reimbursement and the Linkage of Federal Cost Control Programs*, A Report to the Subcommittee on Oversight and Investigations, Committee on Interstate and Foreign Commerce, U.S. House of Representatives (May 1977) (processed), pp. 17–20.

20. William Dowling, "Prospective Reimbursement," *Inquiry* 11 (September 1976): 166.

21. Clifton R. Gauss and Fred J. Hellinger, "Results of Hospital Prospective Reimbursement in the United States," a paper presented to the International Conference on Policies for the Containment of Health Care Costs and Expenditures, Fogarty International Center, June 3, 1976.

22. Washington State Hospital Commission, Proposal to the Social Security Administration for funding of a Prospective Reimbursement Demonstration Project under authority of sec. 222 of P.L. 92–603, 1976 (HCFA Contract No. 600–76–0170).

23. "Hospitals Headlines," *Hospitals* 51 (October 1,1977): 20.

24. Gauss and Hellinger, "Hospital Prospective Reimbursement."

25. U.S. Congress, House, *Voluntary Hospital Cost Containment Act*, H. Rept. No. 95–1789, Part I, p. 37.

26. Carol M. McCarthy, "Prospective Reimbursement As An Impetus to Cost Containment," *Inquiry* 12 (December 1975): 320–329.

27. Paul N. Worthington, "Prospective Reimbursement of Hospitals to Promote Efficiency: New Jersey," *Inquiry* 13 (September 1976): 302–308.

28. U.S. Congress, House, *Voluntary Hospital Cost Containment Act*, H. Rept. No. 95–1789, Part I, p. 37.

29. Ludwig Lobe, Chairman, and Frank Baker, Executive Director, Washington State Hospital Commission, Letter to the Honorable Tim Lee Carter, February 3, 1978 (used with permission).

30. Health Insurance Association of America, "Hospital Cost Control—The State Option," a position paper (December 21, 1977) (processed).

31. Lobe and Baker, Letter.

32. Health Insurance Association of America, "Hospital Cost Control—The State Option," *HIAA Viewpoint* (March 1978) (pamphlet).

33. American Hospital Association, "Revision to Proposed Guidelines for State-Level Review and Approval of Budgets for Health Care Institutions," Resolution approved by the Board of Trustees of the Association January 1978 and by the House of Delegates February 1978.

34. David Salkever and Thomas Bice, "Impact of State Certificate of Need Laws on Health Care Costs and Utilization," *Research Digest Series* (Washington, D.C.: Department of Health, Education, and Welfare, Public Health Service, Health Resources Administration, National Center for Health Services Research, 1977).

35. Ibid.

36. Congressional Budget Office, *Expenditures for Health Care*, p. 33.

37. U.S. General Accounting Office, *Status of the Implementation of the National Health Planning and Resources Development Act of 1974* (Washington, D.C.: U.S. General Accounting Office, 1978), p. 28.

38. U.S. Congress, *The National Health Planning and Resources Development Act*, P.L. 93-641, 93rd Cong., 2d sess., 1974, sec. 1501 (b) (1). See U.S. Government, Federal Register, *Code of Federal Regulations 42*, Part 121, September 23, 1977.

39. Honorable Joseph A. Califano, Jr., Secretary of Health, Education, and Welfare, Letter to Honorable Tim Lee Carter, M.C. (December 1977) (used with permission).

40. U.S. Congress, House, Honorable Paul Rogers, 29 November 1977, *Congressional Record* 123: H12482.

41. U.S. Congress, House, Honorable Abraham Kazen, 29 November 1977, *Congressional Record,* 123: H12483.

42. Symond R. Gottlieb et al., *Reduction of Excess Hospital Capacity: A Suggested Strategy for Action* (Detroit: Greater Detroit Area Hospital Council, Inc., 1977) (processed).

43. Victor M. Zink, "Greater Effort Needed to Control Costs," *Hospitals* 50 (March 16, 1976): 65-67.

44. Sylvia Porter, "Your Money's Worth," copyright 1979, Field Enterprises, Inc. Courtesy of Field Newspaper Syndicate.

45. Michael J. Goran et al., "The PSRO Hospital Review System," *Medical Care* 13 (supplement) (April 1975): 1-33.

46. American Hospital Association, *Washington Developments* 6 (December 28, 1977): 1.

47. See U.S. Congress, House, Committee on Interstate and Foreign Commerce, *Professional Standards Review Organizations: Present Status and Future Prospects*, by Richard B. Burford et al., Comm. Print No. 95-16 (Washington, D.C.: U.S. Government Printing Office, 1977), p. 9.

48. U.S. Department of Health, Education, and Welfare, Public Health Service, Health Services Administration, Office of Planning, Evaluation, and Legislation, *PSRO: An Evaluation of Professional Standards Review Organizations*, vol. 1 (draft) (Washington, D.C.: Health Services Administration, 1977), p. 41. See also Institute of Medicine, *Assessing Quality in*

Health Care: An Evaluation (Washington, D.C.: National Academy of Sciences, 1976).

49. U.S. Department of Health, Education, and Welfare, *PSRO: An Evaluation,* p. 140.

50. Paul Bonner, "On-Site Utilization Review: An Evaluation of the Impact on Utilization Patterns and Expenditures" (Sc.D. dissertation, Harvard School of Public Health, 1976) cited in Congressional Budget Office, *Expenditures for Health Care,* p. 37.

51. Robert Brook and Kathleen Williams, *An Evaluation of New Mexico Peer Review* (The Rand Corporation, 1976) cited in Congressional Budget Office, *Expenditures for Health Care,* p. 37.

52. Kenneth A. Platt, Medical Director of Colorado Foundation for Medical Care, Statement before the U.S. Congress, House, Committee on Interstate and Foreign Commerce, Subcommittee on Health and the Environment, 94th Cong., 2d sess., 1976, cited in Congressional Budget Office, *Expenditures for Health Care,* p. 37.

53. Institute of Medicine, *Assessing Quality.*

54. U.S. Department of Health, Education, and Welfare, *PSRO: An Evaluation,* p. 92.

55. Congressional Budget Office, *Expenditures for Health Care,* p. 36.

56. See U.S. Department of Health, Education, and Welfare, Public Health Service, Health Resources Administration, *Health: United States 1976–1977* (Washington, D.C.: U.S. Government Printing Office, 1977), pp. 159, 160, 162, 166, 168–179.

57. American Hospital Association, *Hospital Statistics,* 1977 ed., pp. xvi–xvii.

58. Abernethy et al., *Prospective Reimbursement.*

Chapter 5

1. Honorable Jimmy Carter, President of the United States, Message to Congress of April 25, 1977, *Weekly Compilation of Presidential Documents* 13 (May 2, 1977): 604.

2. Ibid.

3. Ibid.

4. Honorable Joseph A. Califano, Secretary of Health, Education, and Welfare quoted in "Hospital Costs: Carter Calls for Controls," *Congressional Quarterly Weekly Report* 35 (April 30, 1977): 788.

5. U.S. Congress, House, Committee on Ways and Means, Subcommittee on Health and Committee on Interstate and Foreign Commerce, Subcommittee on Health and the Environment, *President's Hospital Cost Containment Proposal, Joint Hearings on H.R. 6575,* 95th Cong., 1st sess., 1977, p. 13.

6. Ibid., p. 14.

7. U.S. Department of Health, Education, and Welfare, "Hospital Cost Containment Act of 1977," *HEW News* (press release) (April 25, 1977) (processed).

8. Ibid.
9. Honorable Jimmy Carter, President of the United States, State of the Union Address of January 19, 1978, *Weekly Compilation of Presidential Documents* 14 (January 23, 1978): 93.
10. U.S. Congress, House, *Joint Hearings on H.R. 6575*, p. 14.
11. Herman Somers quoted in "Hospitals Headlines," *Hospitals* 57 (February 16, 1977): 17–18.
12. U.S. Department of Health, Education, and Welfare, Office of the Deputy Assistant Secretary for Planning and Evaluation/Health, September 1977.
13. Ibid.
14. P. Joseph Philip, "New AHA Indexes Provide Fairer View of Rising Costs," *Hospitals* 51 (July 16, 1977): 175–182.
15. U.S. Congress, House, Honorable Tim Lee Carter, 15 July 1977, *Congressional Record* 123: E4532.
16. See U.S. Congress, House, *Joint Hearings on H.R. 6575*, Material submitted for the record by the Department of Health, Education, and Welfare on "Empirical Research on Hospital Cost Functions," pp. 127–130.
17. U.S. Congress, Senate, Committee on Human Resources, Subcommittee on Health and Scientific Research, *Hospital Cost Containment Act of 1977, Hearings on S. 1391,* 95th Cong., 1st sess., 1977, p. 237.
18. Ibid., p. 50.
19. Joseph Eichenholz, Office of the Assistant Secretary for Health, Department of Health, Education, and Welfare, Personal Communication. June 5, 1977.
20. Milton Roemer and Max Shain, *Hospital Utilization Under Insurance* (Chicago: American Hospital Association, 1950).
21. U.S. Department of Health, Education, and Welfare, "Justification of the $2.5 Billion Capital Expenditure Ceiling," Briefing Document provided to the Committee on Interstate and Foreign Commerce, Subcommittee on Health and the Environment during consideration of H.R. 6575, August 1977 (processed).

Chapter 6

1. U.S. Congress, House, Committee on Ways and Means, Subcommittee on Health and Committee on Interstate and Foreign Commerce, Subcommittee on Health and the Environment, *President's Hospital Cost Containment Proposal, Joint Hearings on H.R. 6575, 95th Cong., 1st sess.,* 1977, p. 657.
2. Ibid., p. 262.
3. Executive Office of the President, Council on Wage and Price Stability, *The Rapid Rise of Hospital Costs*, by Martin Feldstein and Amy Taylor, Staff Report January 1977 (Washington, D.C.: U.S. Government Printing office, 1977).
4. U.S. Congress, House, *Joint Hearings on H.R. 6575*, p. 663.
5. Ibid.

6. U.S. Department of Health, Education, and Welfare, Office of the Assistant Secretary for Legislation, "Hospital Cost Containment: A Summary of Legislation Pending Before the House of Representatives," a briefing paper supplied to members of Congress, March 13, 1978 (processed).

7. U.S. Congress, Senate, Committee on Human Resources, Subcommittee on Health and Scientific Research, *Hospital Cost Containment Act of 1977, Hearings on S. 1391,* 95th Cong., 1st sess., 1977, p. 167.

8. Ibid., p. 168.

9. U.S. Congress, House, *Joint Hearings on H.R. 6575*, p. 135.

10. Stuart Shapiro, M.D. quoted in John K. Iglehart, "The Hospital Lobby is Suffering from Self-Inflicted Wounds," *National Journal* 9 (October 1, 1977): 1530.

11. John Alexander McMahon quoted in Iglehart, *"The Hospital Lobby,"* p. 1530.

12. Iglehart, *"The Hospital Lobby,* p. 1530.

13. Ibid.

14. U.S. Congress, House, *Joint Hearings on H.R. 6575*, p. 263.

15. Ibid, p. 270.

16. U.S. Congress, Senate, *Hearings on S. 1391*, p. 257.

17. U.S. Congress, House, *Joint Hearings on H.R. 6575*, p. 300.

18. Ibid. pp. 593–594.

19. Ibid., p. 774.

20. U.S. Congress, Senate, Committee on Finance, Subcommittee on Health, *Medicare-Medicaid Administrative and Reimbursement Reform Act, Hearings on S. 1470*, 95th Cong., 1st sess., 1977, p. 191.

21. U.S. Congress, House, *Joint Hearings on H.R. 6575,* pp. 540–541.

22. Paul Feldstein in National Council of Community Hospitals, *A Reference Report on Hospital Cost Containment* (Washington, D.C.: By the Author, 1977), p. 23.

23. U.S. Congress, House, *Joint Hearings on H.R. 6575*, p. 545.

24. Ibid., p. 693.

25. Ibid., p. 694.

26. Ibid., pp. 1156–1158.

27. Ibid., pp. 620–625.

28. Ibid., pp. 628–633.

29. Ibid., p. 723.

30. Ibid., p. 307.

31. Ibid., pp. 334–335.

32. U.S. Congress, Senate, *Hearings on S. 1391*, p. 231.

33. U.S. Congress, House, *Joint Hearings on H.R. 6575*, p. 332.

34. U.S. Congress, Senate, *Hearings on S. 1391*, p. 232.

35. Ibid., p. 609.

36. Executive Office of the President, Council on Wage and Price Stability, *Hospital Costs* by Feldstein and Taylor.

37. U.S. Congress, Senate, *Hearings on S. 1391*, p. 429.

38. Ibid., pp. 598–599.

39. Ibid., p. 616.
40. Ibid., p. 710.
41. Ibid., pp. 701–702.
42. Ibid., pp. 704–705.
43. Ibid., p. 245.
44. See Inglehart, "The Hospital Lobby," p. 1529.
45. U.S. Congress, Senate, *Hearings on S. 1391*, p. 245.
46. Ibid., pp. 237–238.

Chapter 7

1. U.S. Congress, House, Honorable Paul Rogers, 30 June 1977, *Congressional Record* 123: E4281.
2. U.S. Congress, House, Committee on Interstate and Foreign Commerce, Subcommittee on Health and the Environment, *Hospital Cost Containment Act of 1977, Hearings on H.R. 8121 and H.R. 6575*, 95th Cong., 1st sess., 1977, p. 117.
3. Ibid., p. 179.
4. Blue Cross Association, Letter to the Honorable Tim Lee Carter, August 15, 1977 (used with permission).
5. U.S. Congress, House, *Hearings on H.R. 8121 and H.R. 6575*, p. 104.
6. Ibid., pp. 179–180.
7. Ibid., p. 165.
8. Ibid., p. 114.
9. U.S. Congress, House, Honorable Dan Rostenkowski, 14 July 1977, *Congressional Record* 123: H7161–H7165.
10. U.S. Congress, House, *Hearings on H.R. 8121 and H.R. 6575*, p. 123.
11. U.S. Department of Health, Education, and Welfare, Office of the Deputy Assistant Secretary for Planning and Evaluation/Health, "Percentage Increase in Inpatient Expense Per Admission for Community Hospitals," reproduced in U.S. Congress, House, Committee on Interstate and Foreign Commerce, *Summary of H.R. 6575, As Reported by the Subcommittee on Health and the Environment*, Comm. Print No. 95-35, 95th Cong., 2d sess., 1978, pp. 38–39.
12. American Hospital Association, *Hospital Statistics*, 1978 ed.
13. U.S. Congress, House, Honorable Tim Lee Carter, 15 July 1977, *Congressional Record* 123: E4532.
14. Ibid.
15. U.S. Congress, Senate, Honorable Richard Schweiker, 1 July 1977, *Congressional Record* 123: E4220–E4221.
16. Government Research Corporation, *A Proposal for State Rate-Setting: Long-Range Controls on the Cost of Institutional Health Services* (Washington, D.C.: National Journal, May 1977).
17. Honorable Tim Lee Carter, Personal Communication, April 5, 1978.
18. Honorable Tim Lee Carter, Personal Communication, August 10, 1978.
19. U.S. Congress, Senate, Honorable Herman Talmadge, 5 May 1977, *Congressional Record* 123: S7201

20. Honorable Jimmy Carter, Letter to the Honorable Herman Talmadge, as quoted in U.S. Congress, Senate, Committee on Finance, Subcommittee on Health, *Hospital Cost Containment and End Stage Renal Disease Program, Hearings on S. 1391, S. 1470, and H.R. 8423*, 95th Cong., 1st sess., 1977, p.140.
21. Ibid.

Chapter 8

1. David Main, Minority Staff, Subcommittee on Health and Scientific Research of the Committee on Human Resources, U.S. Senate, Personal Communication, September 10, 1977.
2. U.S. Congress, Senate, *A Bill to Establish a Transitional System of Hospital Cost Containment*, S. 1391 as Reported by the Committee on Human Resources, 95th Cong. 1st sess., 1977.
3. U.S. Congress, Senate, Committee on Human Resources, *The Hospital Cost Containment Act of 1977: Summary and Analysis of Consideration*, Comm. Print 95-146, 95th Cong., 1st sess., 1977, p. 59.
4. Harvey Pies, Assistant Minority Counsel, Committee on Ways and Means, U.S. House of Representatives, Personal Communication, July 29, 1977.
5. "Capital Close-Up: Representative James T. Broyhill." *Hospitals* 52 (March 16, 1978): 36.
6. American Health Care Association, Letter to the Honorable Tim Lee Carter, September 19, 1977 (used with permission).
7. Honorable Paul Rogers, "Dear Colleague" letter to the Honorable Tim Lee Carter, October 21, 1977 (used with permission).
8. Michael Hash, Director, Legislative Division, American Hospital Association, Washington, D.C., Personal Communication, October 14, 1977.

Chapter 9

1. Honorable Jimmy Carter, quoted in *C.O.T.H.* (Council on Teaching Hospitals) *Report* 11 (October 1977): 4.
2. U.S. Congress, House, Honorable Dan Rostenkowski, 2 November 1977, *Congressional Record* 123: H12086.
3. The Voluntary Effort, "Actions Approved by the National Steering Committee on Voluntary Cost Containment," a position paper, December 20, 1977 (processed).
4. See John K. Iglehart, "The All-Volunteer Cost Control Plan," *National Journal* 10 (February 11, 1978): 236.
5. John Alexander McMahon, James H. Sammons, M.D. and Michael D. Bromberg, Letter to Chairmen of Hospital Governing Boards, Chief Executive Officers, and Chiefs of Medical Staffs, January 11, 1978. Copies provided to Members of the Subcommittee on Health and the Environment (used with permission).
6. Honorable Dan Rostenkowski, Statement to the House of Delegates, American Hospital Association, Washington, D.C., February 1, 1978.

7. Ibid.
8. Iglehart, "The All-Volunteer Plan," p. 236.
9. Ibid.
10. Elizabeth Wehr, "Hospital Cost Control," *Congressional Quarterly Weekly Report* 36 (March 4, 1978): 595.
11. "Rostenkowski Enlists Support for Cost Containment Bill," *Washington Report on Medicine and Health* 32 (February 20, 1978): 2.
12. Wehr, "Cost Control," p. 596.
13. Idem, "House Committee Scraps President's Hospital Cost Control Proposal," *Congressional Quarterly Weekly Report* 36 (July 22, 1978): 1886.
14. Idem, "Cost Control," p. 1596.
15. Ibid.
16. U.S. Department of Justice, Anti-Trust Division, Letter to the Voluntary Effort, quoted in *C.O.T.H. Report* 12 (June 1978): 3.
17. Peter Libassi, General Counsel, U.S. Department of Health, Education, and Welfare, quoted in *C.O.T.H. Report* 12 (June 1978): 3.
18. John Alexander McMahon, American Hospital Association, quoted in *C.O.T.H. Report* 12 (June 1978): 3.
19. See "FTC's Pertschuk Says Voluntary Effort Raises Serious Anti-Trust Questions," *Washington Report on Medicine and Health* 32 (July 17, 1978): 2.
20. John Alexander McMahon, American Hospital Association, Letter to the Honorable Tim Lee Carter, August 10, 1978 (used with permission).
21. U.S. Department of Labor, Bureau of Labor Statistics, *Consumer Price Index*, August 1978.

Chapter 10

1. "Rostenkowski Enlists Support for Cost Containment Bill," *Washington Report on Medicine and Health* 32 (February 20, 1978): 2.
2. Honorable Paul Rogers, "Dear Colleague" letter to Honorable Tim Lee Carter. May 17, 1978 (used with permission).
3. Ibid.
4. Ibid.
5. See discussion of this controversy in Chapter 4 supra.
6. Michael D. Bromberg, Letter of May 19, 1978; James Sammons, M.D., Letter of May 19, 1978; and Leo Gehrig, M.D., Letter of May 20, 1978 to members of the Committee on Interstate and Foreign Commerce (used with permission).
7. Elizabeth Wehr, "Hospital Cost Control Measure Limps Along," *Congressional Quarterly Weekly Report* 36 (July 15, 1978): 1776.
8. Victor Cohn, "Vote on Hospital Costs Bill Deferred," *Washington Post,* 26 May 1978, p. A4.
9. Honorable Jimmy Carter quoted in Cohn, "Vote Deferred."
10. Honorable James Broyhill and Honorable Edward Madigan, "Dear Colleague" letter to Honorable Tim Lee Carter, June 6, 1978, (used with permission).

11. Honorable James Santini, "Dear Colleague" letter to Honorable Tim Lee Carter, May 26, 1978 (used with permission).
12. Elizabeth Wehr, "Hospital Cost Control Measure Inches Along," *Congressional Quarterly Weekly Report* 36 (June 17, 1978): 1545.
13. Ibid.
14. See Chapter 8, p. 79.
15. Honorable Tim Lee Carter, Statement of June 14, 1978 to the Committee on Interstate and Foreign Commerce, U.S. House of Representatives (typewritten).
16. Wehr, "Measures Inches Along," p. 1546.
17. Honorable Tim Lee Carter, Statement of June 21, 1978 to the Committee on Interstate and Foreign Commerce, U.S. House of Representatives (typewritten).
18. U.S. Department of Health, Education, and Welfare, "Statement of Secretary Joseph Califano," *Press Release* (June 20, 1978) (processed).
19. See Elizabeth Wehr, "Body Blow Dealt to Hospital Cost Bill," *Congressional Quarterly Weekly Report* 36 (June 24, 1978): 1600.
20. See Honorable Dave Stockman, "Supplemental Views," in U.S. Congress, House, *Voluntary Hospital Cost Containment Act of 1978*, H. Rept. No. 95-1789, Part I to Accompany H.R. 6575, 95th Cong., 2d sess., 1978, pp.105-128.
21. Paul Feldstein, An *Empirical Investigation of the Marginal Costs of Hospital Services* (Chicago: University of Chicago Press, 1961).
22. Judith R. Lave and Lester B. Lave, "Hospital Cost Functions," American Economic Review 60 (June 1970), pp. 379-395.
23. Martin Feldstein, *Economic Analysis for Health Service Efficiency,* (Amsterdam: North Holland Publishing Co., 1968), Chapter 5. See also U.S. Congress, House, *Joint Hearings on H.R. 6575,* Material submitted for the record by the U.S. Department of Health, Education, and Welfare on "Empirical Research on Hospital Cost Functions," pp. 127-130.
24. Wehr, "Body Blow," p. 1600.
25. Ibid.
26. Ibid.
27. Dick Warden, Assistant Secretary for Legislation, U.S. Department of Health, Education, and Welfare, Letter to Honorable Tim Lee Carter and other members of the Committee on Interstate and Foreign Commerce, July10, 1978 (used with permission).
28. See David S. Broder, "After the Summit Leadership," *Washington Post,* 23 July 1978, p. C7. See also Carl T. Rowan, "Carter's Still Very Much the Outsider," *Atlanta Constitution,* 26 July 1978, p. 4.
29. Elizabeth Wehr, "House Committee Scraps President's Hospital Cost Control Proposal," *Congressional Quarterly Weekly Report* 36 (July 22, 1978): 1885.
30. U.S. Congress, Senate, Honorable Gaylord Nelson speaking for the Nelson Amendment to H.R. 5285, 12 October 1978, *Congressional Record* 124: S18343.
31. Ibid.

32. U.S. Congress, Senate, Honorable Herman Talmadge speaking for H.R. 5285 as amended by the Committee on Finance, 12 October, 1978 *Congressional Record* 24: S18339.
33. Ibid.
34. Ibid.
35. Ibid.
36. "Carter Would Veto Talmadge Bill," *Washington Report on Medicine and Health* 32 (August 28, 1978): 1.
37. Adapted from U.S. Congress, Senate, *Congressional Record* 124: S18345.
38. "Talmadge Issues Hot Rebuttal to Califano's Criticism of His Bill," *Washington Report on Medicine and Health* 32 (August 28, 1978): 2.
39. U.S. Congress, Senate, Honorable Gaylord Nelson speaking for the Nelson Amendment to H.R. 5285, 12 October 1978, *Congressional Record* 124: S18342.
40. Ibid.
41. Ibid.
42. Ibid.
43. "Talmadge Issues Hot Rebuttal," p. 2.
44. See U.S. Congress, Senate, Honorable Gaylord Nelson, *Congressional Record* 124: S18342.
45. Ibid.
46. Ibid.
47. Ibid., p. S18344.
48. "The Health Scene This Week," *Health Services Information* 5 (October 16, 1978): 1.
49. U.S. Congress, Senate, 12 October 1978, *Congressional Record* 124: S18328–S18409.
50. U.S. Congress, Senate, Honorable Herman Talmadge speaking against the Kennedy Amendment to H.R. 5285 (The Kennedy Amendment is identical to Title I of S. 1391 as amended by the Committee on Human Resources) 12 October 1978, *Congressional Record* 124: S18359.
51. U.S. Congress, Senate, Honorable Gaylord Nelson and Honorable Herman Talmadge in a colloquy, 12 October 1978, *Congressional Record* 124: S18394.
52. U.S. Congress, Senate, Honorable Richard Schweiker speaking against the Nelson Amendment to H.R. 5285, 12 October 1978, *Congressional Record* 124: S1839.
53. See Art Pine, "Carter Wants a No-Growth Budget, Sparing Pentagon," *Washington Post*, 6 November 1978, p. A2.

Chapter 11

1. Honorable Walter Mondale, Vice President of the United States, in *Controlling Health Costs, Conference Proceedings* (Washington, D.C.: National Journal, March 1978), p. 67.

2. Estimate supplied by the U.S. Department of Health, Education, and Welfare, Social Security Administration, Office of the Actuary, 1977.

3. Data supplied by the U.S. Department of Health, Education, and Welfare, Office of the Deputy Assistant Secretary for Planning and Evaluation/Health and is based upon American Hospital Association data, 1977.

4. Ibid.

5. *Washington Developments* 7 (March 28, 1978): 3.

6. Data supplied by the American Hospital Association, Division of Legislation, Washington, D.C., 1977.

7. U.S. Department of Labor, Bureau of Labor Statistics, *Consumer Price Index*, June 1977.

8. Paul Feldstein in National Council of Community Hospitals, *A Reference Report on Hospital Cost Containment* (Washington, D.C.: By the Author, 1977), p. 23.

9. Data supplied by the U.S. Department of Health, Education, and Welfare, Office of the Deputy Assistant Secretary for Planning and Evaluation/Health, 1977.

10. U.S. Department of Health, Education, and Welfare, "Justification of the $2.5 Billion Capital Expenditure Ceiling," Briefing Document provided to the Committee on Interstate and Foreign Commerce, Subcommittee on Health and the Environment during consideration of H.R. 6575, August 1977 (processed).

11. Data supplied by the U.S. Department of Health, Education, and Welfare, Office of the Deputy Assistant Secretary for Planning and Evaluation/Health and is based upon American Hospital Association data, 1977.

12. Ibid.

13. U.S. Department of Health, Education, and Welfare Office of the Assistant Secretary for Legislation, "Hospital Cost Containment: A Summary of Legislation Pending Before the House of Representatives," a briefing paper supplied to members of Congress, March 13, 1978 (processed).

14. John Alexander McMahon, James H. Sammons, M.D., and Michael D. Bromberg, Letter to the Chairmen of Hospital Governing Boards, Chief Executive Officers, and Chiefs of Medical Staffs, January 11, 1978. Copies provided to members of the Subcommittee on Health and Environment (used with permission).

15. Honorable Joseph A. Califano, Jr. Secretary of Health, Education, and Welfare, quoted in American Enterprise Institute for Public Policy Research, *Proposals for the Reduction of Hospital Costs* (Washington, D.C.: American Enterprise Institute, June 1978), pp. 45–48.

16. American Enterprise Institute, *Proposals*.

17. "Hospital Hoodwink," *Congress Today* 4 (April, 1978): 16.

18. "A Plan for Closer Physician Involvement," *AMA Newsletter* 10 (March 13, 1978): 1. Reprinted with permission of the American Medical Association.

Index